HEALTH CARE
MELTDOWN

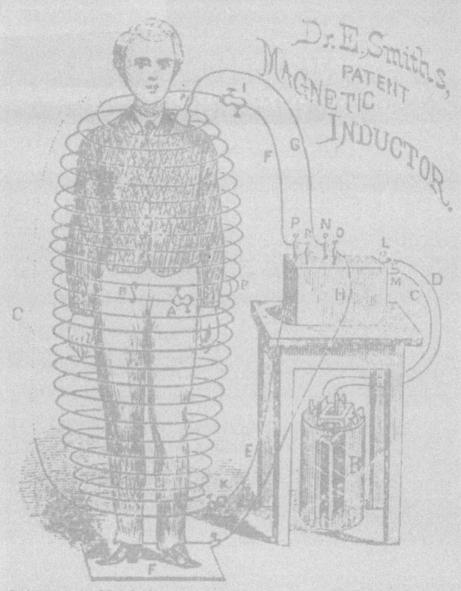

Dr. E. Smith's,
PATENT
MAGNETIC
INDUCTOR.

HEALTH CARE MELTDOWN

CONFRONTING THE MYTHS AND FIXING OUR FAILING SYSTEM

Robert H. LeBow, MD

Foreword and new chapters by

C. Rocky White, MD

Alan C. Hood & Company, Inc.
CHAMBERSBURG, PENNSYLVANIA
2007

The patent medicine illustrations in the book were printed on mailing envelopes, a popular advertising device in the 19th century. The original envelopes are a part of the postal history collection of Bob LeBow.

The cures were peddled to the public by a group sometimes referred to as *snake oil merchants*, who created a mythology of misinformation in order to enhance their own economic interests.

Manufactured in the United States of America

Published by Alan C. Hood & Co., Inc.
P. O. Box 775, Chambersburg, PA 17201

Library of Congress cataloging-in-publication data

LeBow, Robert H., 1940-
   Health care meltdown : confronting the myths and fixing our failing system
/ Robert H. LeBow ; foreword and new chapters by C. Rocky White. -- [Rev.
ed.].
      p. ; cm.
   Includes bibliographical references and index.
   ISBN-13: 978-0-911469-30-1 (pbk.)
   1. Medical care--United States--Evaluation. 2. Medical policy--United
States--Evaluation. 3. Social medicine--United States. 4. Medicine--United
States. I. White, C. Rocky, 1961- II. Title.
   [DNLM: 1. Delivery of Health Care--economics--United States. 2. Delivery
of Health Care--trends--United States. 3. Health Policy--United States. 4.
Medically Uninsured--United States. W 84 AA1 L449h 2007]
   RA395.A3L413 2007
   362.10973--dc22

                                                            2007019815

Dedicated to the memory of
TERRY REILLY,
my partner in the struggle for
Health Care for All

* * *
* *
*

Publisher's Note

Shortly after the first edition of *Health Care Meltdown* arrived from the printer, Dr. Bob LeBow suffered a catastrophic cycling accident that left him totally paralyzed. In late 2003, Bob died of complications arising from his injuries and was never able to continue his crusade for universal health care.

Last year his widow, Gail LeBow, and I agreed that the health care situation Bob had described so well in 2002 had only gotten worse, and Bob's book needed updating and revision with an eye toward influencing the 2008 U.S. presidential campaign. Gail pointed me in the direction of Dr. Rocky White, who readily agreed to take on the task.

With Rocky's revisions and contributions, the editorial expertise of Jo-Ann Kachigian, and the help of many other dedicated people, this 2007 edition of *Health Care Meltdown* addresses the continuing failure of America's health care financing system and demonstrates how a single-payer approach can restore fairness and sanity to health care in the United States of America.

Alan C. Hood
April 2007

Contents

Part One: The Problem
A Wasteful, Dysfunctional System
and a Nation Kept Clueless

Part Two: Toward Finding a Solution

Foreword

As I SLOWLY CLOSED THE DOOR TO MY OFFICE OF IO YEARS, the darkness quietly filled the room like the sadness that filled my heart. The lock clicked shut, finalizing the chapter of what I felt at the time was a personal failure of enormous magnitude. I walked down the hallway cluttered with boxes and packing paper, handed in my key, and stepped through the back door into the light of uncertainty and what former Colorado Governor Richard Lamm called "The Brave New World of Health Care."

As a simple country boy growing up on the plains of Nebraska, my only aspirations were to follow in the footsteps of generations of farmers and ranchers. Instead, I've taken a long, convoluted—and miraculous—journey that has led me to become a leader in health care reform.

While my small-town, agricultural background and fundamentalist, evangelical upbringing would shape my conservative Republican political views, ultimately, they would also be the catalyst for a more progressive ideology molded by a love of the land and the simple people who live there.

After farming and working at various agriculture-related jobs for a couple of years after high school graduation, I found myself, through the hand of God, attending a small Bible school in Oklahoma (the heart of the Bible belt). I then went on to earn a bachelor's degree at the University of Nebraska, where I completed medical school and my residency, and ultimately achieved board certification in internal medicine.

As the first in my family to attend college, let alone graduate from medical school, I found myself in 1994 a country doctor and the only internist in the Nebraska panhandle outside of Scottsbluff. Seeking camaraderie and a shared call schedule with other internists, my road turned again to a remote rural area in south-central Colorado called the San Luis Valley, with the central medical hub located in Alamosa.

After arriving there in the spring of 1996, I joined a private, fee-for-service, for-profit multi-specialty group consisting of internal medicine, pediatrics, and family practice, along with general surgery, orthopedics, ENT, ophthalmology, and ob/gyn.

At that time, there were 11 full-time practicing internists throughout the Valley with a full staff of five in our group. It remained that way for several years. Little did I know that by January 2005 I would be the only full-time practicing internist left in the entire Valley. In fact, between 1996 and September 2004 (when our group closed its doors), 35 partners had come and gone—and 26 of those were primary care physicians.

In that same time span, we went from a vital, profitable organization of more than 20 partners to a beleaguered, bloodshot, battle-weary band of 8 who had made a pact to take the high ground, circle the wagons, and hold to the last man.

It would have been easier to cut and run and look for greener pastures. But, as you will experience through the chapters of this extraordinary book, for the medical profession and the patients it serves, there are no greener pastures.

Our group began to see trouble on the horizon in the late 1990s. At first, our group was no different from any other across the country, with the usual decreasing reimbursement in the face of ever-increasing overhead. Our initial response was typical— rewrite the compensation formula and start working smarter, not just harder. Little did we know that we were simply rearranging the deck chairs on the Titanic.

With the ushering in of a new millennium, we began to experience our own personal "health care meltdown." From the late 1990s to 2004, health care inflation was raging from 10 to 12 percent a year, with Medicaid and Medicare reimbursements essentially remaining flat or actually decreasing. Only small incremental increases were seen in insurance payments.

But what was to me the most alarming and detrimental change was the accelerating number of hard-working, middle-class people who either could not afford to keep their health insurance or, in order to save on cost, were moving to policies with fewer benefits and higher deductibles and co-pays.

As we later discuss in greater detail, the two great design flaws of the market-driven philosophy encompassed by high-deductible plans and health savings accounts (HSAs) are: (1) the majority of middle-class Americans cannot afford to make financially meaningful contributions to theirs, let alone pay for their insurance premiums, and when they do need to access the health care system, they often delay care, thus making their condition worse on presentation; and (2) they oftentimes are unable to meet the obligations of those $2,500 or $5,000 or, in some instances, $10,000 deductibles. Guess who has to eat the loss?

While patients then have to choose between making payments to doctors and hospitals for their deductibles or continuing to pay monthly premiums for the increasingly poor insurance coverage, physicians and hospitals are forced to try and collect the huge first dollar expenditures and many times end up writing them off.

In our case, the uncollectable accounts receivables continued to climb. This, in conjunction with a highly saturated population of Medicare and Medicaid patients, eventually broke us.

Through it all, the profits of the insurance industry have soared.

The point of no return for us personally came in 2004. As the collapse of our clinic became imminent, those who chose to stay behind approached the local hospital. The hospital had to either buy us out or lose the only surgical and specialty care it had. What choice did any of us have? We couldn't stay in business, and without us the community would lose the only surgical and specialty services it had for over 5,000 square miles. It was a shotgun wedding—not a move to gain market share, but one of mutual survival. Thankfully, for the time being, it has been successful (or relatively so). The hospital (a nonprofit entity) manages, so far, to operate on a slim 1.5 percent margin, but even in the 2005 fiscal year, it still lost $600,000 on the clinic. Why?

Simply put, when we see a Medicaid patient, we lose 30 cents on the dollar. When we see a Medicare patient, we barely break even. Of our clinic population, 23 percent is Medicaid and 28 percent is Medicare.

The uninsured rate in the San Luis Valley is close to 24 percent (nearly 50 percent higher than the state or national average). As a result, you can imagine the number of poverty-stricken patients that we end up seeing as "self pay" (a euphemism for the uninsured) and almost always an uncollectable debt.

With these types of demographics and with health care inflation continuing to surge at two to three times the growth of our economy, it doesn't take a PhD in economics to realize that the health care system in our region and many similar places across America is unsustainable.

Now, as a conservative Republican who has always held an entrepreneurial "pull yourself up by your own bootstraps" free-market philosophy, you can imagine the frustration I began to experience while trying to provide compassionate, quality health care in the context of a market in which the accustomed rules of business economics don't apply. I understood intimately how to run a practice. I was the executive secretary for the Board of Directors for the clinic for several years, helping to make the day-to-day decisions of running a multimillion-dollar clinic. I also was the medical director for an HMO insurance company.

But I knew little, if anything, about the big picture of state and federal health care policy and how this nation managed to get itself into such a mess.

So, beginning in the summer of 2002, I began to study in the evening when I came home from the clinic. For months I voraciously devoured any literature or books I could get my hands on that had anything to do with health care policy and finance. Bit by bit, I began to piece the puzzle together and was shocked and dismayed by what I found.

I then took the knowledge that I gathered, along with my years of experience as a full-time practicing physician, and said, "Okay, if our system is really this screwed up, what could we do to fix it?"

Again, more laborious study, market analysis and cost comparison, potential quality outcomes, patient access issues, and demographics were rolled through every conceivable scenario of reform. No matter how I turned the cube, the answer never changed. That answer was nearly impossible for me, a free-market Republican, to accept. Two points became painfully clear:

1. Until we remove the motive of profit from the financing of health care, we cannot and we will not resolve our current health care crisis.

2. Any group that proposes reform policy that maintains the use of for-profit insurance companies in a so-called free market is being driven by one single motive—to protect the golden coffers of their share of the $2 trillion cash cow!

To continue down this road is paramount to suggesting that we privatize our fire and police services and turn them into for-profit organizations. You do that and people will die—just like they are dying now under our current health care system!

Needless to say, this revelation shook my old-line Republican values. After all, this is America, and there is nothing wrong with profit and making money, is there?

Yes, there is, when it comes at the expense of human life.

At that time, I was unaware that there were many others who had come to the same conclusion. So I started to write a book (and had actually written several chapters). I was discussing my findings one afternoon with a fairly liberal colleague of mine, believing that my more conservative colleagues would probably think I had gone over the edge. She asked me if I'd ever heard of a group called Physicians for a National Health Plan (PNHP) and directed me to their Web site. I couldn't believe it! They actually had come to the same conclusions that I had! Little did I know that some of them had been pushing for this type of reform for decades!

So, in the following spring, I attended a leadership conference in Chicago sponsored by the PNHP. It was there that I was introduced to a book called *Health Care Meltdown* by Dr. Bob LeBow. As I started to read it, I was absolutely floored. This guy had written my book!

Bob's experiences and writing style were so similar to mine, and even the chapters were like mine. At that point, I decided that working on my book was redundant since it had 'already been written.' So I refocused my energies, went on the speaking trail, and encouraged others to read *Health Care Meltdown*.

In December 2005, I was invited to speak at the PNHP annual national meeting in Philadelphia. Bobbie Dennett, a health activist from Bob LeBow's hometown (Boise, Idaho) heard me speak and invited me to come to Idaho to speak on health care reform. She thought I might appeal to the more conservative constituency represented in Idaho. I accepted her offer, and she returned to Boise to share the news with a health care reform group of which Bob LeBow's wife, Gail, was a part.

Tragically, a few years earlier, in 2002, Bob had been critically injured in a cycling accident just one week after his book was first published; he eventually died in 2003 of complications from his injuries. When I accepted the offer to come to Idaho, neither Bobbie Dennett, Gail LeBow, nor anyone else for that matter had known about my story or the book I had never finished.

Early in 2006, publisher Alan Hood wanted to run a second edition of *Health Care Meltdown* with updated data in time for the 2008 election cycle; he wondered if Gail LeBow had anyone in mind. Knowing only a little about me and certainly nothing of my history, she said, "Yes, I do." And the rest, as they say, is history.

And so, it is with great honor that I present to you the updated and second edition of the book I never wrote, by the man I never met, with the story that Bob LeBow never had the chance to finish.

I am sure you will find it not only inspiring, revealing, and even shocking, but that when all is said and done, you will be as convinced as I am that the economic principles of a free market are designed for only one purpose—to maximize profits. This is America, and there is nothing wrong with those principles as they apply to business. But ensuring the health of our nation is not a business, and we must stop treating it as such. Until we have the courage to remove the profit motive from the financing of health care and implement some form of a single-payer system that has the authority to contain cost and is accountable to the people, we will not be able to stop the impending "Health Care Meltdown."

C. Rocky White, MD
Alamosa, Colorado
November 2006

Prologue

THIRTY YEARS AGO, as I was heading toward a career in international health, I became aware of how poorly our American health care system was working. I saw how millions of our own people were being denied the care they needed. And I began to appreciate how those same people were being robbed of their dignity.

In 1971 I had completed a 2-year stint as a U.S. Peace Corps physician in Bolivia, and the following year I finished a master's in Public Health course in international health at Johns Hopkins. It was then that I decided to switch my geographic focus and work with our own "third world" right here in America.

I moved my family to Idaho to join a migrant health center that had just received its initial grant and became its first medical director. In an old grocery store that had been purchased for $6,000, and in a variety of makeshift venues like church basements, I helped organize and run a series of health centers that served poor people, then largely migrant farmworkers, in southwest Idaho. Mostly, I took care of patients. As a family practitioner, I did everything from obstetrics to geriatrics. Over 30 years I delivered almost 2,000 babies. I've followed some of the same patients for three decades, long enough to deliver babies for women I'd help to bring into the world 20 years earlier. And I've helped to train scores of health care professionals, including nurse practitioners, physician assistants, medical students, and residents.

In the mid-'80s I began to wonder about what I was doing. Despite all the sleep deprivation I could handle, my patients and I were still hitting the same stone wall when it came to dealing with our health care system. Despite all our efforts as a "safety-net" community health center, people were still forced to go without needed care. They were still being robbed of their dignity. I was still having to "beg, borrow, and steal" to get care for my patients. And I came to the realization that change was not going to come unless our nation changed how it looked at health care and at ourselves as a nation. Americans were not going to regain their dignity unless our nation changed.

It was a personal tragedy that inspired me, directly and indirectly, to become a health care activist. In 1986 my younger son, Tommy, died at age 16 in an auto accident. He might have survived if he had been wearing his seat belt. Without exaggerating, I calculated that I had told him to put his seat belt on at least 2,000 times. A month after his death, the Idaho State Legislature was holding hearings on a new seat belt law for Idaho. I testified before committees in both the House and the Senate. The law would not have passed had I not spoken up. It passed the House by only three votes, and I received letters from three representatives who said they changed their vote because of my testimony.

As a result of my son's untimely death, through a series of unusual circumstances, I also became a columnist for our local newspaper, now *The Idaho Press-Tribune*. I kept that job for 8 years, and I wrote a column every week—any subject I wanted, at $6 a column—except when I was campaigning for political office.

More poignantly, with Tommy's death there was also a more personal feeling that motivated me to become an activist. I felt responsible to do whatever I could to help others avoid the kind of sorrow and grief that comes with, for example, the death of a child.

Inspired to enter politics to change the raw deal my patients were getting with their health care, I ran for a House seat in the Idaho State Legislature—three times. I picked the wrong party to win, but I learned a lot about politics. In one election campaign, I knocked on the doors of close to 3,000 households. And I got to listen to the gripes of a lot of people. In 1988 I became active with Physicians for a National Health Program (PNHP), a national organization striving for universal coverage through national health insurance. For 2 years, in 1998 and 1999, I was president of that organization.

While I continue to work at my community health center in Idaho, since January 2001 I've become a half-time "health care activist." Like many of my fellow activists, I spend long hours preparing and making presentations to a variety of groups, planning initiatives, organizing and attending meetings, writing articles, and generally trying to drum up support for universal coverage for health care. In my quest, I've found that one of the greatest obstacles to meaningful health care reform is the degree to which we Americans are clueless about our health care system. Most Americans—including politicians and even knowledgeable health care professionals who should know better—have been led down an assortment of primrose paths. They have been sucked into arguing about the fine points of a variety of diversions, such as the nearly irrelevant "patient protection" debate. They have even been led to give serious consideration to options that would make our disaster of a health system even more complex and unresponsive.

I see my patients continuing to wander in the health care wilderness, without much hope of finding the path out. Even more ominous, I see millions of currently insured Americans facing the danger of losing their coverage—and their dignity—as our health care system slips towards "meltdown." The options I see being proposed offer a few crumbs to my patients and increasing obstacles for everyone else, but no lasting solution. And I see these options being justified by the usual host of myths that have been used for decades to derail meaningful health care reform.

Until we can confront the myths and choose a real solution that provides affordable, comprehensive health care for every person in America, an ever-increasing number of middle-class Americans will join my low-income patients in health care limbo. Middle-class folks' misadventures with health care will increasingly resemble the stories of the uninsured and underinsured that I have related in this book. Middle-class Americans are already quietly acquiescing to a growing number of indignities foisted upon them by our failing system. And they are learning to accept the type of rationing endured by my uninsured patients: health care that is delayed or skipped altogether. As we approach another crossroads for our American health care system, I fear that more and more Americans will suffer unnecessary pain and illness, as well as increasing humiliation.

I am passionate on the issues because my passion is rekindled on a daily basis as I struggle with my patients to jump through unnecessary and wasteful hoops to meet their health care needs. I have tried to remain objective in what I describe. However, I have deliberately strayed from an academic approach because, in dealing with the problems involved in health care reform, I am trying to concentrate more on some of the deeper and more human dimensions that are not addressed in the usual academic or economic studies.

I have drawn many examples from my Idaho experience, where I have been practicing for many years. If anything, the situation for health care is worse elsewhere, especially in large urban areas where the indignities can be perpetrated with more anonymity. Idaho remains a small state where personal connections still count, and Idaho has had the good fortune of being largely passed over by the "managed-care revolution." But even in Idaho, I'm seeing the increasing burden being laid upon middle-class people, people with insurance, insurance that is becoming progressively more inadequate.

This book is an attempt to bring to light some of the myths that are obstructing change and to propose a solution so that every person in America (including my patients) can get the health care he or she needs. In this richest of all countries, we have the resources, both economic and human, to change the quagmire that our health care system has become. What we lack is the vision, the political will, and the courage to stand up to the vested interests.

Bob LeBow, MD, MPH
Boise, Idaho
July 2002

Acknowledgments

I WANT TO THANK PROFUSELY those people who laboriously plowed through early draft versions of this book. Without their help, this work would not have been possible. Their advice and direction have been invaluable. I am especially grateful to Marcia Bondy, Ed Crawford, Maria Eschen, Ellen Kurnit, David Reese, Julia Robinson, and Todd Swanson for their perseverance in giving me enlightened feedback. To my brother, Joel LeBow, I owe a special thanks, for reading the whole draft document at a single sitting, and then getting back to me with insightful comments from a consumer's point of view.

I also owe special thanks to my wife of 40 years, Gail, who has provided ongoing critical suggestions as well as unwavering support for this project. Thanks also go to my "technical support" team, including Jennifer LeBow, Nicole LeFavour, and Jean Miller.

With respect to the issue of health care in America, and my involvement in the "cause" of Health Care for All, I'd like to thank Don McCanne, for his informative e-mail network "Quote of the Day," which has provided many useful leads; Physicians for a National Health Program, which has supplied a host of useful data and information; the late Terry Reilly, who recruited me in 1972 to work with migrant farmworkers in Idaho; his wife, Rosie Delgadillo Reilly, who, for more than 30 years, has been a champion of the underserved; colleagues in my practice, who have provided me with "stories of the uninsured and underinsured"; innumerable other colleagues, all involved in the "cause" as well, who have provided me with thought-provoking ideas and inspiration; and my patients, who have been gracious enough to share their experiences and ideas with me.

—Bob LeBow, MD, MPH

I WOULD LIKE TO EXPRESS SPECIAL THANKS to the following people who contributed so enormously in helping to make this second edition a reality. First, Gail LeBow, who had the faith in me to continue Bob's work; Bobbie Dennett, who brought us together; Russ Johnson and Gwen Heller, at the San Luis Valley Regional Medical Center, who have given me the freedom to advance the cause of health care for all; and Jo-Ann Kachigian, for her meticulous wordsmithing. Special gratitude is extended to John Geyman, for updating the references; Don McCanne, my brother in arms, who keeps us sharp and vigilant; Ida Hellander, who helps maintain our focus; and Quentin Young, who carried the torch before I was even born!

I am grateful for my mother, Maxine White, who gives me strength with her prayers, and for my daughters, Ariel and Aleeya, who so often must patiently share their daddy with the rest of the world. But my deepest and heartfelt thanks go out to my lovely and talented wife, Debbie, with whom I will celebrate 20 glorious years of marriage as the second edition of this book hits the press. Without her patient support and inspiration, this work, along with all the other hair-brained projects I get involved in, would never be possible. Deb, no matter how high I fly, you truly are the wind beneath my wings.

C. Rocky White, MD

Confronting the Myths:
Can America Halt the Slide Toward
Health Care Meltdown?

Rigoberto sat nervously on the edge of the exam table and broke into tears. A large and reserved 17-year-old, he had asthma and a nasty cough that hadn't improved in 2 weeks. I was about to prescribe an inhaler and antibiotics. "What's wrong?" I asked. He glanced at his mother. "On our way here, I found out we didn't have money to pay for the visit," he said, wiping his eyes with the back of his hand.

I reassured him that, since we were a community health center, money wasn't a problem. I forewarned our pharmacy to give him the prescriptions without pressing for payment. But after I left the exam room, our collections person entered and politely asked for $8, our "nominal" fee. Mother and son broke into tears of embarrassment and left without the medications.

AMERICAN HEALTH CARE is once again at a "crossroads," one of several windows of opportunity for change that we have had over the past 90 years. The last "opportunity moment" in American health care—marked by President Clinton's ill-fated and ill-conceived "managed-competition" proposal—ended in 1994 with the collapse of his plan. Since then, we have had a vacuum in leadership and direction. "Market" principles and the pursuit of profit have become the norm for health care. Cost shifting from employers to employees has accelerated, and access to care has become more difficult. The number of uninsured Americans has grown and now, with the economic downturn, is increasing even more. America's brief "managed-care revolution," with its temporary slowing of some health care costs, is dead. The American public would no longer put up with being exploited and abused by managed-care organizations. As for the uninsured, their situation has only become worse.

As we approach this new crossroads for health care, our system is failing and in imminent danger of collapse or "meltdown." Fortunately, for the moment, the system is still capable of meeting the health care needs of many who find themselves in a crisis. We have wonderful technology. There are thousands of dedicated and caring clinicians and others who try their best to help people in need. But more and more, the needs of people are not being met. The number of Americans without adequate access to care is growing. More and more, Americans are delaying care or going without needed services. They show up at a crisis stage in increasingly beleaguered emergency rooms.

Hospitals are overcrowded and understaffed. Over 90 percent of our nursing homes have an inadequate number of nurses. Ambulances circle around waiting for an open spot at an emergency room. Medical errors happen much too frequently. Costs are soaring. Patient expectations are soaring too, as new technologies and drugs become available. Waste abounds as money that could be used for patient care is instead diverted to pay for higher administrative costs that are a result of the increasing (and unnecessary) complexity and "gaming" of our system. Our federal programs, Medicare and Medicaid, are endangered. There is no planning, no vision for the future, as our nonsystem seems to be imploding.

Millions of Americans, the 46 million without health insurance, have been deprived of their dignity, and we're in danger of losing our dignity as a nation. America is the only developed nation that fails to guarantee access to needed care for all its citizens and the only advanced country that permits someone to go bankrupt because of poor health. Even Americans who have health insurance are increasingly being squeezed or sometimes forced to forgo care, as depicted somewhat melodramatically in the recent movie "John Q." A survey done at the end of 2001 showed that 43 percent of Americans with private insurance feared that their family's insurance coverage might be eliminated or reduced in the next year.[1]

Millions of Americans have become "health care beggars."[2] Millions more, including middle-class Americans, are at risk of joining them as beggars in the near future as the cost of health care soars.

Our Poor Performance and Perverse Incentives

DESPITE OUR STANDING AS the richest country in the world—and despite our spending nearly twice as much per person on health care than any other country—the overall results have been disappointing, dehumanizing, and at times even abysmal. Our health status indicators rank us near the bottom among the developed countries in such measures as life expectancy and infant mortality. In 2000 the World Health Organization ranked the U.S. health care system at number 37 overall.

Meanwhile, our population grows more obese and sedentary. Substance abuse continues at a high rate. Failure to deal adequately with mental health has contributed to our burgeoning prison population. And debt from health care is now the second highest reason for personal bankruptcy. The pursuit of profit has assumed primacy over the pursuit of what is best for people.

Why the disconnect? Where have we failed? Does anybody care?

Our health care system—or, more precisely, nonsystem—has evolved into a monster, a disorganized, overly complex creature that robs people of their health, their money, and their dignity. Yet the great majority of Americans are unaware—or clueless—of what has happened to America's health care. Blind belief in certain icons of American economic theory—icons that have limited relevance to health care—have helped cause our current dilemma.

Faith in "the market" and competition, stress on "personal responsibility" and individualism, and dislike of government regulation or managed anything have contributed to the creation of a system that turns a blind eye to millions of patients like Rigoberto who "do without." We Americans live in a milieu of purposeful health care ignorance. Merchants of misinformation and myth spend millions of dollars to keep us clueless. By doing so, they limit improvements in our health care system to piecemeal bits of change. Remember Harry and Louise? The bus from Canada? Citizens for a Better Medicare? They're only a few of the scams perpetrated on the American public by the vested interests. By delaying or averting a comprehensive solution, the health care entrepreneurs prolong the time they are able to reap profits from the system. Profits they keep for themselves and their shareholders, while my patients, and millions more like them, are forced to become "health care beggars" or "go without."

A large part of our problem stems from the perverse incentives of the system. For much too long, America's health care system has been driven (on the supply side) by self-interest. Instead of commitment to community and cooperation, the overriding ethic of health care in America has become self-interest and the pursuit of profit. The American people have been left out of the equation. Even worse, they have been systematically duped and then blamed for being "overutilizers" by some of the same special-interest groups that misled them. Americans are told to exercise more "personal responsibility," a code word for shifting costs to the consumer. But they have been set up by the health care industry (insurers, drug companies, medical establishment) to have high expectations and to create a demand for expensive goods and services. As for the people who can't afford the expensive services, they don't matter. There are no profits to be made from the poor, unless they can qualify for a government program that will pay their bills.

The Search for a Comprehensive Solution

AN INTEREST IN UNIVERSAL COVERAGE once again seems to be growing, though it appears to be morphing into a less ambitious goal of "reducing the number" of the uninsured. Some of the factors creating pressure for health care reform include an economic recession, a growing unemployment rate, and the accelerating costs of health care. Health insurance premium rates rose by 11 percent in 2001 and were expected to rise 15 percent in 2002. The events of 9/11 also may have reawakened some sense of community in America as well as a questioning of the axiom that less government is always better. There is also a growing sense of despair from the ever-increasing number of Americans who are hurting from being *under*insured. Including the 46 million uninsured Americans, we are reaching perhaps a critical mass of people, a total of maybe as many as 90 million (not even including Medicare beneficiaries), who need help. With the growing number of people in distress, including many more middle-class Americans, there is bound to be a more strident demand for change.

Groups (such as the insurance industry, the pharmaceutical companies, and some elements of the medical care establishment) with special financial interests in our health care system will likely continue to play games of disinformation to derail significant change. And they will twist the mantra of "personal responsibility" to make people believe that financial barriers to care, like increased deductibles and co-pays, are good for them. They will invoke the "mantra" of "socialized medicine" to attack any increased role for government. Yet government needs to have a role—at the very least in oversight, coordination, and leadership—if we are to fix our failing health care system.

We are hearing increasingly about incremental or "piecemeal" reforms, about vouchers, tax credits, health savings accounts (HSAs), and "defined contributions" from employers. There is now a plethora of ideas about how to "cover more Americans." Most of them are complex, and some experts argue that we may have to make our system more complex than it already is. But people who have been working within the system, and who appreciate the abuses and loss of dignity suffered by so many Americans seeking adequate health care, know these "piecemeal" solutions will only prolong the agony and maintain the status quo. And the status quo has become increasingly intolerable as our system heads toward meltdown.

Getting America Clued In

I'VE WRITTEN THIS BOOK in an effort to shed light on the degree of cluelessness that permeates American health care. I have attempted to use my 30 years of experience working within a dysfunctional health system and my efforts as a health care activist to sort out the realities and the myths. I am concerned that the "piecemeal" direction in which we seem to be headed will not help *my* patients or the millions of other Americans who are likely to join their ranks as "health care beggars." I worry that even friendly allies who advocate for "doing something" will compromise the chances for millions of Americans to get the health care they need. If even a few million Americans are left hanging in limbo, our nation will not have regained its dignity.

I have not included lengthy economic analyses. Instead, I have provided a selective bibliography that readers can refer to for more detailed information. I have tried to concentrate on an analysis of the key issues that we must address to achieve meaningful reform. I have also attempted to provide an *ad hoc* type of road map for reaching the goal. Some of the principal themes that I address in this book include:

- The high degree of misinformation and myth that has been intentionally used by what I have termed the "modern-day snake oil merchants" to hawk their products and discredit system changes that might limit their influence or profits.

- The twisted "market" model as it has been applied to health care. How, instead of putting the customer first, it has in fact put the patient last.

- How the "personal responsibility" mantra and co-pays/deductibles act as barriers to care and are used to "blame the victims" and shift cost or increase profits.

- How we need to think more in terms of societal or community responsibility.

- A smattering of real patient experiences: misadventures

of the uninsured and the underinsured. (All the names have been changed.)

- How Americans have missed the boat on prevention and what we must do about it.

- Affordability, and the poor value we get for our health care investment in America, especially compared to other developed nations.

- What direction do we need to take at this crossroads? How can we arrive at a solution that is really universal and affordable and provides *everyone* with the health care they need?

- The importance of "one risk pool"—and not lip service to "pluralism"—in reaching a universal coverage that is fair and affordable and does not exclude the sick.

- Some humility in admitting that health care alone cannot give America good health, that it takes a wider approach involving social and economic change, including efforts at prevention, to reach good health.

- That Health Care for All is a key first step in returning dignity to individuals, families, and our nation, and that, without it, we will be unable to resolve the gaping health disparities that we have in America today.

"One Risk Pool"/ National Health Insurance

I BELIEVE THAT UNLESS America chooses a solution that incorporates the concept of "one risk pool," such as national health insurance, we will never solve our dilemma. Former Senator Bob Kerrey expressed his support for this approach when he testified before the Senate Finance Committee in March 2002.[3] He advised against adding a prescription drug benefit to Medicare— "not unless you are prepared to make fundamental changes in the way Americans finance the cost of their health care." He went on to assert:

"Beginning with a universal entitlement does not mean higher spending or more governmental interference with the choices made by patients or providers. In truth, it could mean a lot less of both. It would mean that we would start thinking about ourselves as a single group of 280 million Americans who are all part of the same health system and who all need to face the challenge of matching our appetite for quality with our capacity to pay."

Perhaps there are solutions other than national health insurance—or its equivalent—for America to achieve universal coverage in a way that is both comprehensive and affordable. It's possible that we could model a solution after approaches adopted by some European countries and express the goal as "assuring universal access to care for all needed medical services." However, as described in the chapters that follow, it is difficult to imagine how there could be a fairer, more efficient approach than "one risk pool" that would truly cover *every* person in America. The type of solution envisaged in this book is embodied in this concept. "One risk pool" is virtually synonymous with what is referred to as a "single-payer" approach, though they are not precisely the same since "one risk pool" refers more to the group of people covered as opposed to a payment mechanism.

Under "one risk pool" (see the Appendix for a brief summary of "frequently asked questions" about "one risk pool") everybody in America would be covered in the same health insurance plan. There would be no questions about enrollment or eligibility. Since the largest possible number of people would be "pooled together," there would be economies of scale. There would be no more "cherry-picking," no more excluding of the poor or the sick from access to needed care. No one would go bankrupt because of medical bills. Savings from the elimination of middlemen and other administrative costs would allow every person coverage with a comprehensive package of benefits without increasing our overall spending on health care.

Instead of premiums, co-pays, and deductibles, the plan would be funded through progressive taxation and would have a trust fund specifically devoted to the plan, much like today's Medicare. There would be a larger government role in collecting the taxes and overseeing the plan. But the delivery system would remain predominantly private, as it is today. Each person would be able to choose any provider of services he or she chose, in effect *increasing* choice. "One risk pool" refers to the financing mechanism only, has no direct effect on the delivery system, and does not in any way diminish the role of the private sector in providing health care. It is not socialized medicine. It is a way to minimize administrative costs and create equity.

The general principles that comprise this approach, which would in effect be a form of national health insurance, include the following:

- *True universality. Everybody in, nobody out, with one risk pool. No more "cherry-picking," or exclusion of high-risk people from coverage.*

- *Tax-based financing, like Medicare, in accordance with income, instead of premiums, deductibles, and co-pays. Not free care, since everybody pays into the system through taxes.*

- *Full choice of providers in a delivery system that remains a mix of private and public. Not socialized medicine, but national health insurance in the same way Medicare is a national insurance program.*

- *Elimination of the odd link between employers and health insurance coverage.*

- *Coverage for all necessary services, including inpatient and outpatient care, emergency care, long-term care, mental health, treatment for substance abuse, prescriptions, and basic dental and eye care with no discrimination by type of illness or ability to pay.*

- *True integration of public health and preventive services with adequate funding, both on a personal and community basis.*

- *Continued funding for the special services necessary to serve special population groups; for example, immigrants, migrant farm workers, and the disabled.*

- *The practice of medicine based on scientific principles.*

- *A national trust fund dedicated specifically to health care.*

- *National planning that allows a high degree of local autonomy. A national health board with regional or state-by-state equivalents.*

- *Public accountability. Eliminates the "opaque"(hard to fathom) financing practices of the current system.*

- *Global budgeting, which entails setting priorities, but is flexible enough to support medical education, research, and excellence in medicine.*

- *Simplified administration with greatly reduced administrative costs, leaving 90 to 95 percent of health care funds for patient care, prevention, and research.*

- *Reasonable and equitable reimbursement for health care providers.*

- *Insurance companies would be allowed to sell policies only for uncovered services.*

- *Treatment of health as a "public good" instead of as a market commodity.*

PART ONE

The Problem

A Wasteful, Dysfunctional System and a Nation Kept Clueless

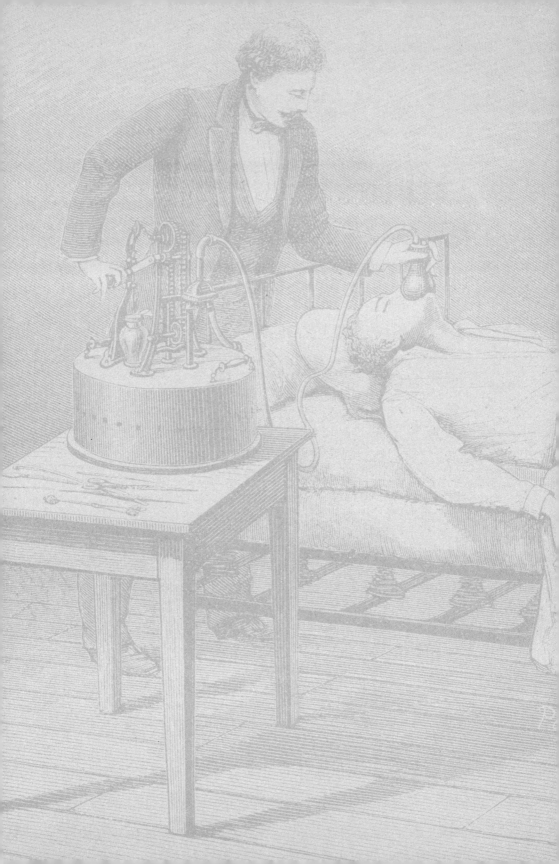

Chapter 1

Myths, Misinformation, and the Pursuit of Profit

"This country has the best health care system in the world."
—President George W. Bush

"That's strange; I thought Mr. Bush and I lived in the same country."
—C. Rocky White, MD (interview excerpt, Montana Public Radio, January 2006)

IN THE ANTHOLOGY OF MYTHS about health care in America, there is the "Alpha Myth" that asserts "America has the best health care system in the world." It is heard over and over, most frequently from the mouths of politicians. Many Americans, not knowing any better, believe it. This and a host of other myths about health care in America have arisen partly out of ignorance and partly from our insularity.

There is a national sentiment that (of course) America must be the best in almost everything. So it is with health care. Playing on Americans' assumption of superiority, special interests with major financial stakes in our health care sector have made certain to reinforce and spread the mantra that we have "the best health care system in the world." The more the American people can be lulled into accepting this mantra, the more the special interests can continue to exploit the system to their own advantage and profit.

Facts belie these myths, however. As Stephen Bezruchka,[1] Barbara Starfield[2] and others have pointed out, the United States does very poorly when it comes to the standard measurements of health status. In fact, we rank about 20th or lower when compared with other developed nations in such measures as life expectancy, infant mortality, and immunizations.

Much of this disparity comes from the ever-widening gap in America between the rich and the poor. Bezruchka even theorizes that the wide gap itself is the reason for the differences. America has a higher percentage of people living in poverty than most other developed countries. And America, unlike all the other developed countries, has not embraced the principle that health care should be a basic human right. In America, health care is a privilege, not a right.

The 2000 World Health Organization (WHO) report on the world's health care systems ranked the United States 37th "overall." In fact, we tied Fiji at 54th in "fairness" as it applies to the way a country treats its citizens within its prospective health care system. The United States has done little to improve its standings according to the latest WHO report from 2005. Our report card is abysmal: life expectancy, 27th; maternal mortality, 29th; infant mortality, 35th; overall mortality ages 15 to 60, 35th; odds of dying before age 5, 36th; population over age 60, 40th. In fact, the United States leads the world in only two categories: amount of money spent on health care per capita per year (now over $7,000) and the amount of that money spent as a percentage of our gross national product (165 percent). We have the world's best technology, which Americans can access if they are able to pay for it. However, we also are unique in having a fragmented, inefficient, and administratively wasteful system that excludes 1 out of 6 Americans from insurance coverage.

A Myriad of Myths

BESIDES THE FALSE MANTRA that "America has the best health care system in the world," there are many other oft-cited myths about health care in America. These are used to promote a variety of political or economic agendas. They include but are not limited to:

1. We don't have a problem with access to care in America since anyone can get needed health care by going to an emergency room.

2. The system's not broken, so it doesn't need to be fixed.

3. "The market" can solve the problems with our health care system.

4. Private solutions are always better than public solutions.

5. Medicare is going broke.

6. America can't afford universal coverage.

7. Americans will not accept health care "rationing" like they have in other countries.

8. Canada's health care system is terrible and failing.

9. The insured are subsidizing the care of the uninsured.

10. We don't have the resources to handle the increased demand for services that would result from universal coverage.

11. Drug prices are higher in the United States because our pharmaceutical industry spends billions of dollars on research and development.

12. We can get to universal coverage through incremental or piecemeal change.

13. Americans will never accept a "single-payer" system.

Myth #1: Everybody Has Access to Care Through the Emergency Room

WE DON'T HAVE A PROBLEM with access to care in America since anyone can get needed health care by going to an emergency room (ER). Unfortunately, way too many Americans are forced to use ERs to obtain their health care. Many people, especially the uninsured, lack a regular health care provider and have nowhere else to go. But the ER is the most expensive and inefficient way to deliver primary care.

For example, consider a person with a urinary tract infection or bronchitis. Going to the ER instead of a primary care provider often ends up with a 2- to 4-hour wait and a bill for $500. If that person had gone to a primary care clinician, it probably would have been an hour wait and a bill closer to $80. Moreover, the ER physician usually does not know the patient, has no previous medical records, and is much more obliged to practice defensive medicine (that is, more expensive, with more tests). Follow-up is incomplete and uncertain. The patient is often given a few sample pills and a prescription to take to a pharmacy only to find they can't afford to buy the medicine.

Emergency rooms are being stressed to the maximum. *USA Today* published a front-page story[4] about how the ERs in the United States were falling apart under the strain of too many patients. This scenario now plays out each winter (the season for high patient demand) at many ERs in cities throughout America.

ERs are being inappropriately used for primary care in America because our system to deliver primary care is inadequate. Only in recent years has there been an increase in outpatient "urgent care" or "doc-in-the-box" clinics offering extended hours of service. However, these types of clinics deal only with immediate problems, they lack continuity of care, and typically are not available in the poor urban, inner city, and remote rural areas.

We saw a young uninsured woman who had gone to one of these clinics for a severe kidney infection. She was treated appropriately, given a shot of an antibiotic, and a prescription for Cipro. She bought the Cipro for $129 but 2 days later still was not feeling better. It turned out that her infection was resistant to Cipro but sensitive to Septra, an $8 medicine. She was concerned that she wouldn't be able to afford the cheaper medicine because she only had $2 left after paying for the Cipro. Fortunately, we were able to give her what she needed.

A particularly disingenuous myth related to the "access to care through the ER" myth is that, since anyone can get care through an ER, the uninsured in America are in fact not suffering adverse effects to their health. The data to the contrary are overwhelming. They are summarized in a report released in 2000 by the American College of Physicians-American Society of Internal Medicine: "No Health Insurance? It's Enough to Make You Sick—Scientific Research Linking the Lack of Health Coverage to Poor Health."[5]

The Kaiser Commission on Medicaid and the Uninsured came out with a similar report in May 2002. Entitled "Sicker and Poorer: The Consequences of Being Uninsured," their report documents how being uninsured *does* matter. Through an extensive literature search, they show (among other findings) that the uninsured: (1) have a 10 to 15 percent higher mortality rate; and (2) earn 10 to 30 percent less because of their poor health.[6] Also, in May 2002, the Institute of Medicine released the second of a series of six reports on the consequences of uninsurance. Entitled *Care Without Coverage: Too Little, Too Late*, the study estimates that more than 18,000 adults die each year in the United States because of the lack of health insurance.[7]

Myth #2: We Don't Need to Fix What's Not Broken

THE SYSTEM'S NOT BROKEN, so it doesn't need to be fixed. A favorite theme of some right-wing pundits is to deny that America has a health care crisis. This line of rhetoric assumes that the system must be functioning well since it works for 85 or 90 percent of Americans. It is still true that, for people with good health insurance and good connections to our health care system, the quality of the care they receive can be excellent. In an opinion piece that appeared in *American Medical News,* Richard F. Corlin, MD, the president of the American Medical Association (AMA), extolled the medical care he received when he was traveling and suffered a collapsed lung. He concluded that, ". . . Most of our health delivery system is working very well and should not be discarded under the guise of correcting the problems of the uninsured or any other aspects of health care that need our attention."[8]

He's partially correct—and lucky. Many of our caregivers are competent and dedicated. But we have major problems with medical errors, poor access to care, the failure to practice scientific-based medicine, and the lack of a preventive approach to health care. However, it's primarily the financing system, and every aspect that relates to that system, that's failing. And the financing of health care drives the delivery system. In any given year, the great majority of Americans experience only minimal interface with our system. For example, the healthiest 20 percent of Americans spend only about $14 a year on health care. They have little to complain about, so they can be included in the "satisfied" category. But there are many millions of Americans who are not so healthy and, unlike Dr. Corlin, do not have good insurance or the savvy to work a system that can be very complex and frustrating.

We're failing the most with the uninsured, the 15 percent of Americans for whom the system does *not* work. Add to that number the additional 50 million or so Americans who are *under*insured. These two groups of people often are the ones who need the care the most. They include many people with chronic diseases and "preexisting conditions" who are unable to afford insurance. Many of the uninsured don't even bother to show up for care unless they're critically ill. They are the "invisible uninsured."[9, 10] Can our society really accept a "margin of error" of 15 percent or more when the result is serious disability or death? That's what we're doing today with health care. We're playing Russian roulette with the lives of the uninsured and, increasingly, the *under*insured.

Myth #3: "The Market" Is the Solution

"THE MARKET" CAN SOLVE THE PROBLEMS with our health care system. Americans are led to believe that faith in "the market" is the American way and that, given a chance, "the market" can solve anything. However, since the demise of the Clinton Plan in 1994 and the leadership vacuum that followed, we've had a chance to see what the market could do for health care.

With respect to the financing of health care, "the market" has been an abject failure. The market may work well with automobiles, housing, and fast food. But buying health care is a far cry from buying a hamburger. The much-vaunted advantage of market "competition" in health care has only resulted in increased woes for providers and patients. With competition being almost exclusively based on cost, the result has been the creation of oligopolies, the control of the market by large corporations.

Although managed care did lead to a temporary flattening of health care cost inflation, the effect was short-lived. It was mostly due to cutting back on provider reimbursements and denying care to patients. Managed-care organizations underpriced their products to gain market share and, as a result, many of them lost money in the late '90s. That is not the case today! Moreover, the popular backlash to the abuses of managed care forced managed-care organizations to abandon many of their rationing mechanisms. Maybe the forces of competition could lead to better outcomes if quality were the issue, but with cost and profits as the motivators, "the market" in health care has led to:

- An increase in the number of uninsured. There has been a dramatic increase in the number of uninsured over the last 20 years, despite periods of strong economic growth. The uninsured rate in this country now exceeds 46 million. With our current economic slowdown resulting from the 9/11 aftershock, dramatic increases in energy prices, and the war in Iraq, more than 3,200 Americans a day are being added to the rolls of the uninsured!

- Despite rhetoric to the contrary, we saw a marked decrease in choice, as opposed to other developed countries where choice has been increasing.

- Markedly increased diversion of resources to administration, marketing, and profits, with less money left for patient care. Overall administrative costs in the United States are now estimated at 25 to 30 percent, with the highest rates being in areas where the "penetration" of managed care is the highest.

- A decrease in the quality of care and an increase in medical errors as cost saving became the main priority.

- A failure to deal with some of the more pressing—but less profitable—aspects of health care, such as mental health and public health. The failure to fund public health adequately became particularly evident when our nation was recently faced with the anthrax scare and now, more recently, the shortage of flu vaccines. This aspect of the failure of "the market" is extensively discussed in a book by Laurie Garrett.[11]

- An expansion of for-profit HMOs, a phenomenon that has come to be almost as reviled as the tobacco industry in America.

- Millions of dissatisfied Americans.

- Frustrated physicians because administrative demands have limited the amount of time they are able to spend with patients.

Myth #4: Private Is Always Better Than Public

PRIVATE SOLUTIONS ARE ALWAYS BETTER than public solutions. Discrediting government has become (for some, at least) a popular American sport, along with (for some health care providers) ripping off government health care programs. Keeping the anti-government myth alive (for example, "You don't want the government in your medicine cabinet, do you?") is an important element in maintaining control for a private sector that has excelled at manipulating regulations to maximize profits, as the pharmaceutical and energy (Enron, for example) industries have done.

There is a subgroup of physicians—some would have us believe they are more numerous than they actually are—who are fiercely anti-government. In the July 2001 issue of *Physician's Money Digest*, the editor summed up their position on health care. He asserted that, "Most sensible physicians believe the key to correcting our health care trouble is to empower patients and physicians and to remove government interference." The patient counterpart for these "sensible" physicians might be the famous Florida senior who, during the campaign debates about the future of Medicare, angrily declared, "I don't want the government messing with my Medicare!" There is a love-hate relationship here. Seniors overwhelmingly support Medicare, yet there is a conflict in American society over the role of government.

Meanwhile, robbing our major governmental health insurance programs, Medicaid and Medicare, through up-coding, unnecessary expensive services, or just plain fraud has led to huge fines. Tenet paid $300 million, HCA/Columbia $740 million, and Blue Cross of Illinois $140 million for overcharging Medicare and Medicaid. Not long ago there was an outcry that Medicare was so inefficient that it had lost $23 billion in overpayments. Yet someone had to bill Medicare. The blame belongs with the (mostly private) health care providers who were systematically (and often fraudulently) overbilling.

Government does have an appropriate role in many functions and does, in fact, do some things right. The events following the September 11 terrorist attacks may have in fact tempered the lack of trust in government. Suddenly, the American public was looking to government for leadership. And the federal government, with the public's blessing, is actually assuming a function formerly done by the private sector: airport security. Other examples of public sector responsibility accepted by the public are defense, road construction, public safety, public education, and the regulation of essential utilities.

A recent example belying the myth that "private is always better" was the deregulation of the power industry. Many people were hurt by the ensuing chaos in energy prices. Americans found themselves exploited by entrepreneurs who maximized their opportunities for profits in the name of the "free market." The debacle was capped by the Enron disaster and recent revelations about how Enron manipulated energy prices. The same phenomenon, though perhaps not quite as obvious, has been happening to health care in America.

When we look at the administrative cost and profit-taking of the insurance industry, which it euphemistically refers to as "the medical loss ratio," the comparison between the public and private sectors is not even close. Though it is hard to generalize on the overhead costs for private-sector health insurance, generally it varies between 9 and 30 percent, about 15 percent on the average. These private insurance costs contribute in a major way to the global administrative cost of health care in America—a cost estimated at about 25 percent by Richard Huber, the ex-CEO of Aetna/US Healthcare. Health economist J. D. Kleinke has drawn attention to an even more egregious overhead cost in the private sector: the 50,000 health insurance brokers, or "parasitic middlemen." He estimates they collect commissions that range from 3 to 20 percent of the total cost of insurance plans, adding hundreds of billions of dollars to premium costs.[12]

In contrast, Medicare's overhead is only between 2 and 3 percent, and Medicaid (though it varies from state to state) only spends about 5 or 6 percent. Some hospital administrators would argue that the bureaucratic regulations put on providers by Medicare actually make their overheads much higher, but many of these same administrators will agree that in the past decade the bureaucratic demands from the private sector (HMOs, etc.) have been just as onerous, if not more.

I queried Thomas Scully, the former administrator of the Centers for Medicare & Medicaid Services (CMS), about why, at a hearing in October 2001, he had scoffed at the comparative (private versus Medicare) overhead issue. His reply, via e-mail:

> *"Many make that argument—but I don't agree. We are a blind check-writing machine with two percent overhead. A well-run private insurer has 10-12 percent overhead but has far more understanding of its providers and of patient behavior. The program payments are far less efficiently tracked and targeted . . . . Good insurers are far better at spending money and incentivizing good behavior."*[13]

I assume Mr. Scully was referring to the issue of how money is spent. But there is a huge difference between 2 percent and 10 to 12 percent. I suspect that if Medicare, with its economies of scale, had even 1 percent more to spend to assure the money is spent wisely, it could come up to Mr. Scully's standards. As to incentivizing good behavior, we are on different wavelengths. I described to him my experience with insurers in Idaho. Medicare (as of March 2002), through its contractor Pro-West, had helped

27 health clinics in Idaho to set up a computer-generated preventive screening program. This system provides a detailed reminder sheet at each visit for every Medicare patient. In the case of our clinic (we were the first), they spent thousands of dollars to help us set up a database, which also includes every diabetic patient (about 1,000). The result has been greatly improved care for our patients.[14]

In contrast, all I hear from Idaho's premier private insurer is episodic advice on the cost of pharmaceuticals and an occasional clinical education piece that I've already read in a medical journal. There are different kinds of incentives, and "government" often is far superior to the private sector when it comes to prevention.

People have a false impression that Medicare has a bloated bureaucracy. The opposite is actually true. Many of the alleged bureaucratic problems with Medicare have come about because of inadequate staffing—partly as a result of employment freezes—at what used to be called the Health Care Financing Administration (HCFA) and is now CMS. As for the much-disparaged thousands of pages of Medicare regulations, I have been in practice for more than 30 years and have yet to read (or felt the necessity to read) even one of these pages. I've probably had good advice from the office staff, and I once even had some charts audited by Medicare (I passed).

The "bottom line" for patient care is that money spent on administration, overhead, marketing, inflated CEO salaries, and corporate profits is money that cannot be spent on patient care. On this "bottom line"—the Veterans Administration notwithstanding, it's a very specialized example—most government programs, including Medicare and Medicaid, far outperform their private counterparts. Moreover, government programs, unlike the private sector, cannot select out the enrollees to avoid the poor, the sick, or the expensive cases.

Government can be ponderous and slow, but at least people have the opportunity to change what they feel is unfair or wrong through the ballot box or by applying public pressure. In contrast, patients have little or no ability to influence the policies of investor-owned giants such as UnitedHealthcare or Aetna, especially in our current situation where it is primarily employers who purchase the insurance for health care. And, unfortunately, America's current political system gives corporate lobbyists an advantage over the public in influencing government policy decisions.

Myth #5: Medicare Is Going Broke

MEDICARE IS GOING BROKE. I testified about Medicare before a House subcommittee in Washington in 1994 as part of an "expert" panel. I was reflecting on the future of Medicare from the point of view of the National Rural Health Association. Each Republican on the subcommittee made a point of asking each panelist—I'm sure for the record—whether we thought Medicare, if unchanged, was in danger of running out of money. It reminded me of a lawyer trying to make a point for a jury. "Medicare in Crisis" is a political game that has been going on for many years. Obviously, changes will always have to be made—and have been made as necessary in the past—to keep Medicare solvent. Some of the bluster evaporated from the rhetoric when, after the Balanced Budget Amendment (BBA) of 1997, the costs of Medicare in 1999 actually *decreased* by 2 percent. Suddenly, Medicare's solvency got pushed forward by a few decades. And in 2002, the General Accounting Office (renamed the General Accountability Office in 2004), much to the chagrin of some Republicans, extended the solvency date of Medicare to 2030.

The real political agenda behind the "crisis" has been, and continues to be, the privatization, or even the dismantling, of Medicare. The forces of privatization keep alive the myth of "Medicare is going broke" for the express purpose of scaring the American people into believing that Medicare should be "saved" by privatization.

Times have changed since Medicare began in 1965. Although Medicare benefits have evolved somewhat, such as new added benefits to cover more preventive measures and (more recently) Alzheimer's disease, a growing elderly population and new technologies have made the program much more costly. The demographic bubble of the aging "baby boomers" will present a new challenge when this group starts to turn 65 in 2011.

Interestingly enough, overall medical costs were steadily going up when Medicare spending decreased 2 percent in 1999. Perhaps some of the BBA changes that caused this drop were draconian (such as with home health and hospitals). But the savings for Medicare indicated a considerable amount of "working the system," even fraud. And the drop in Medicare costs illustrates that system changes that control costs are possible. Subsequent adjustments in Medicare that corrected some of the overly zealous sections of the BBA illustrate how our political system can be flexible. The ability of the system to respond to needs is evidence that Medicare is not broken but can be changed or fixed without discarding the whole program.

Medicare beneficiaries are overwhelmingly supportive of Medicare. Study after study shows that people want Medicare improved and expanded, not privatized or dismantled. Yet Republicans and a few Democrats, like Senator John Breaux (D-Louisiana), have sought to privatize Medicare. Perhaps they are acting out of a difference in philosophy (a dislike of public programs). Or maybe their actions are influenced by the advice of lobbyists for special-interest groups that see profits to be made in dismantling Medicare.

These same interest groups are responsible for the myth that a privatized Medicare, or Medicare Advantage plans (formerly Medicare+Choice), will offer more choice, while the opposite is true. I have a long-time elderly patient who for years had been followed by a certain ear, nose and throat (ENT) physician for his ear problem. Yet when my patient joined a Medicare HMO (one of the Blues' *Mediwonder* plans, touted by advertisements with smiling seniors on the golf course), he could no longer see the ENT doctor who had done surgery on his ear. He had to go to a new specialist. More choice? The original Medicare offers full choice of any health care provider. Directing Medicare towards managed care (and choice of plans) has only diminished *real* choice.

Yet another hotly contested challenge to our aging population is the skyrocketing cost of prescription medications. Today, pharmaceutical spending is about to surpass physician costs as the second-highest category (behind hospital costs). Medicare beneficiaries are the major users of pharmaceuticals, accounting for more than 40 percent of all drug sales in the United States. The recent Medicare Part D prescription plan holds some promise for relieving seniors of the burden of their medication costs, but the complexity and privatization of the program have raised concern that the most vulnerable of our population (the forgetful, sick, and feeble) may not be able to navigate the bureaucracy to their best interests. Another part of this act, which prohibits the CMS from negotiating directly with the pharmaceutical industry (like the Veterans Administration is able to do), has been felt by some to be a "giveaway" to the drug companies. Medicare's hands have been tied, and it is not allowed to use its market strength to directly leverage drug prices. The privatization theory of allowing competition to contain cost has yet to be borne out. The cost shifting and administrative burden to state Medicaid programs, individual pharmacies, and doctors' offices to implement this program has been monumental. Finally, the price tag of this program far exceeded original projections in an already strained federal budget, and there is no mechanism in place to cap rising drug prices other than an already fragmented and ineffectual "market." With excessive drug company profits protected and a program price tag that promises to strain the federal budget even further, this program promises to be a hotly debated political and economic issue for years to come.

Myth #6: We Can't Afford Universal Coverage

AMERICA CAN'T AFFORD universal coverage. This myth gets reinforcement from those who see personal (or corporate) advantages for continuing the status quo with its opportunities for profits. It plays to the fears of those who feel they already have fairly adequate health care coverage. Examples of these relatively well-off people are certain union groups and retirees. The hypothesis is that if everyone is to be covered, then people who now have fairly good coverage will have to give up or sacrifice some benefits so that there will be enough money to include everyone.

Most Americans do not realize that: (1) every other industrialized developed country assures coverage for everyone; and (2) despite covering everyone, they spend considerably less than we do for health care. The United States spends about twice as much per capita as most industrialized nations. According to the figures from the 2006 World Health Report[15] (2003 last reported calculations using U.S. dollars), per capita spending for health care in the United States was $5,711. Compare this to the next highest industrialized nations—Switzerland at $5,035 and Norway (third most expensive) at $4,976. From there, the numbers challenge us to ask, "What are we doing differently"? $3,204 in Germany, $2,662 in Japan, $2,669 in Canada, and $2,428 in the United Kingdom! Also, according to the report, U.S. health care spending was 15.2 percent of its gross domestic product (GDP) compared with 11.1 percent for Germany, 9.9 percent for Canada, and 8 percent in the United Kingdom. Although comparative figures are unavailable at this time, the most recent numbers released by the Office of the Actuary, Centers for Medicare & Medicaid Services[16] now estimate that in 2006 the United States will exceed $2 trillion in total health care spending. This approaches 16.5 percent of our GDP and places per capita spending at $7,110! And as if that's not depressing enough, they go on to estimate that, by the year 2015, national health expenditures will top $4 trillion and consume 20 percent of our GDP. This will push health care spending to $12,320 per person annually!

These comparative figures sometimes trigger the Alpha Myth (discussed above) that "America has the best health care system in the world" and, of course, the assertion that, "We wouldn't want the type of inferior health care they have in those other countries." This judgment reflects our insularity and ignorance of what actually happens in the other countries. None of the other systems is perfect, and all of them have their problems and their critics, just as we have problems and critics in America. But they do spend a lot less to cover everybody, and their health outcomes are better than ours. Much of the disinformation about other health systems has been disseminated purposefully by organizations such as the AMA.

As for people who live in those other countries (Canada and England, for example), they are often appalled when they hear about how health care works in the United States. The great majority of them wouldn't even consider switching their systems for ours. Of course, there are the exceptions. Access to advanced technology in the United States is a draw to some rich foreigners who come to famous U.S. clinics for their care. Ironically, a great number of Americans who live right here cannot partake of that technology because they can't afford it.

Another interesting argument used by opponents of a national health program has been to point out the migration of Canadian physicians across the border to the United States in order to practice medicine in a more "favorable" climate. According to a recent article in the AMA newsletter, for the first time since the early 1970s the number of Canadian physicians crossing the border and going back to Canada outnumbered those coming south. For the first time in 30 years, it appears that our "favorable climate" has lost its appeal, and as we advance through this study, the reasons will become painfully obvious.

We have such a frightfully wasteful and fragmented health system in the United States—such a complex patchwork of illogical, perverse incentives—that it will be difficult to make the system affordable unless we do basic and significant reform. As discussed above, the estimates vary, but the overall administrative costs of the U.S. system are about 25 to 30 percent. Current estimates of that cost in California, with its terminally developed managed-care systems, run much higher. Tinkering incrementally with the current system, inventing new financial mechanisms such as refundable tax credits, supplemental insurance for all, or health savings accounts (HSAs), will only make the system more complex and more wasteful administratively.

What if we had a system such as an improved Medicare for All, with everyone automatically included? It would be not only fair and just, but would also allow huge administrative savings, at the very least, nearly 30 percent. Health economist Donald Light points out that the overhead of the American health care system is "about three times the overhead in countries with private care but universal access, such as Germany, Japan, and The

Netherlands."[17] Those savings alone, about $400 billion in 2005, would easily cover the costs of insuring every person in America. After all, we already pay for the uninsured in one way or another. A recent article released by Families USA stated that a typical family in the State of Colorado pays approximately $900 per year of its health insurance premiums as a markup to cover the losses of doctors and hospitals that help take care of the uninsured. Without spending one more penny as a nation, we could go a long way toward eliminating the suffering, the pain, and the worry that come from being uninsured or underinsured.

Study after study has shown that universal coverage with a simplified administrative structure, like national health insurance with everyone in "one risk pool," would actually cost us less, while including everybody. From the Congressional Budget Office and General Accounting (now Accountability) Office studies of the early '90s to the more recent state-by-state studies, the single-payer approach has consistently been shown to save money. The most recent studies were done as a part of the state health planning grants funded by the Health Resources Service Administration (HRSA). They showed overall savings of more than 5 percent in both Vermont and California with a single-payer plan that included universal coverage. This type of system with "one risk pool" may be the *only* affordable solution.

What percentage of a country's GDP is appropriate to spend on health care is a whole other (and related) philosophic question. From the viewpoint of corporate America, it seems obscene and uncompetitive that General Motors (on the U.S. side of the border) spends nearly $1,400 for employee health care for every car it produces. But that figure helps bring home the point about perverse incentives. We should be looking at health care from the perspective of the nation as a whole, not just from the point of view of the health care industry. We need to consider breaking the perverse link between employment and health insurance, a link that is not only an accident and unique to America but is also actually hurting U.S. industry by making it less competitive in a world market. The question of how much of our country's GDP we should be spending on health care will be discussed more fully in Chapter 11.

Myth #7: Americans Don't Want "Rationing" of Health Care

AMERICANS WILL NOT ACCEPT health care "rationing" like they have in other countries. "Rationing" is a catchword—like "socialized medicine"—that triggers a series of negative gut reactions. Similar to the way Republicans and Democrats have used the words "death tax" and "estate tax" to mean the same thing, people will argue about whether the time one waits to get a certain procedure done or see a particular doctor should be called "rationing" or "waiting time."

But we already have "rationing" or "waiting times" in America. Maybe Americans don't wait as long to get an MRI or a cardiac catheterization because we have an excess capacity for those kinds of expensive procedures. But how long do we Americans have to wait to get an appointment with an ophthalmologist, an orthopedist, or a lung doctor? My elderly aunt in Chicago who needed a hip replacement had to wait 3 months to see the doctor she wanted. And the chief resident of a Johns Hopkins residency program had to wait almost 3 months for an appointment with a lung specialist. How long would you have to wait to get a physical exam with your family physician? When I asked that question of my HMO in Boston a few years ago, I was told 6 months. Rationing or waiting time?

How about the uninsured? I have a patient who has been waiting several years to have her gallbladder taken out. If she had shown up in the emergency room with a "hot" gallbladder and a temperature of 102°, she would have had it taken out immediately, no questions asked. Of course, as a result, she might have needed to make payments to a collection agency for the next 10 years. But what if her attack hadn't been acute, and her pain and nausea just came back now and then, as is the case with my patient? She'd wait until she became eligible for Medicare at age 65 to get her surgery. I had another uninsured patient with a painful prolapsed uterus who waited about 2 years (until she got Medicare) to get treated. Multiply these patients by a few million to get an idea of the magnitude of the problem we Americans already have with "rationing."

The definition of U.S.-style rationing is: (1) If you can afford it, you can get it; (2) if you can't afford it, you either can't or won't get it unless; (3) it's a dire emergency; and (4) you're lucky enough to catch the problem in time and survive.

Myth #8: We Don't Want Socialized Medicine Like in Canada

CANADA'S HEALTH CARE SYSTEM is terrible and failing. Americans largely dismiss the Canadian system as not worth looking at because the American media campaigns to discredit Canada have been so effective. The United States has a high degree of ignorance about the Canadian system. Even some of my friends who are actively working in health care look down on it. "We don't want Canadian-style health care in America," they say. Often we hear such truisms as, "There are more MRI machines in Houston than there are in all of Canada." Maybe Houston should have fewer.

When I talk about health care reform, I frequently get an array of Canada-bashing type questions—except from the Canadians, who often come up after the session to praise their system and scratch their heads over why the U.S. system is so bad. Canadians are outraged at the hatchet jobs that certain U.S. interest groups (like the AMA and the pharmaceutical industry) have done on the Canadian system. The great majority of Canadians are fiercely proud of their health care system (called medicare with a small "m"). They would not even remotely consider changing it for the American system, which many of them (as well as many Europeans) regard as barbaric.

The Canadian health system has its problems, mostly originating from years of underfunding when a conservative government was in power. There are some waiting times for nonemergency services. Unfortunately, this issue came to a climax in 2005 when a Canadian Supreme Court ruling opened the door for the expansion of private health insurance to allow those who could afford it to effectively pay more for medical services and "jump the queue" of the current system, which in theory would generate more private investment in medical technology. The main reason cited for the ruling was that the provinces had failed to maintain an adequate infrastructure. But personal

communications and studies being done indicate that these waiting times are nowhere near as long or onerous as the critics of the
Canadian system (who call them "rationing") claim. But the
Canadians do have universal coverage with a single-payer system
for each province. No one worries about going without needed
care or about going bankrupt should he/she have a serious illness.
And it's *not* socialized medicine, as the detracting propagandists
would have us believe. The delivery system is overwhelmingly
private. We have much to learn from Canada.[18] The Canadian
system will be discussed further in Chapter 10.

Myth #9: The Insured Pay More to Help Cover the Costs of the Uninsured

THE INSURED ARE SUBSIDIZING the care of the uninsured. This used
to be true, but it's often the opposite today. This myth, and its
opposing counterpart, demonstrates why universal coverage with
"one risk pool" would be fairer. The "cost-shifting" of yesterday,
which was unfair in itself, isn't so simple anymore. Today everybody pays more, but because of the practice of "charge
inflation"—jacking up prices so they can be discounted for health
plans—the uninsured and people with individual insurance are
now substantially subsidizing the care of those with group
insurance plans. "Hospitals, clinics, labs, and physicians charge
individuals [including the uninsured] about four to five times as
much as their regular negotiated fees with the plans and insurers.
[And] insurance companies charge [individuals] much higher
premiums for less coverage on the argument that they are at
serious risk when they insure one person at a time."[19]

The groups most adversely affected by this practice are
Hispanics (the ethnic group with the highest rate of uninsurance,
32 percent in 2000) and immigrants. These practices have been
documented by Consejo de Latinos Unidos, and they are suing
Tenet in a class-action suit for ethnic discrimination.[20]

The largest subsidy to the insured (and not enjoyed by the
uninsured) comes through the tax-free insurance payments made
by employers for employee health insurance. This federal subsidy
for those with employment-based health insurance amounted to

about $140 billion in 2001, or approximately 10 percent of total health care spending. But everyone pays taxes, so the taxes paid by the uninsured, as well as the self-insured, go to pay for health insurance for those with employer-based plans.

The discounts that the managed-care plans have negotiated with hospitals and physician groups mean that the uninsured (and the sheiks) are often the only ones who are now paying full "retail" price.

Of course, some of the uninsured cannot afford to pay, but many do—usually over time and with interest added. On top of being charged several times what the insured are billed, many of the uninsured must also endure the humiliation of being dunned by a collection agency. The poor uninsured person winds up with extra charges and hassles from a collection agency, while the hospital ends up collecting more (even at one-third of the amount billed) from the uninsured person than they would have received from a health plan.

A fall 2000 article[21] in *Health Affairs*, "Gouging the Medically Uninsured: A Tale of Two Bills," describes how the author, who was insured, and her neighbor, who wasn't, paid for their hernia repairs. The uninsured neighbor wound up paying his surgeon (and the hospital) about twice as much for the surgery as did the author, whose HMO had negotiated discount prices with the hospital and physician. I have a low-income uninsured patient, a musician in his forties, who was billed full price (about $2,500) for his hernia repair. He's now paying off his bill to a collection agency—principal plus interest. No wonder the 2000 WHO report ranked the U.S. health care system 54th in the world in "fairness."

The fact that the uninsured, who must fend for themselves in buying health care, actually pay more for their care than the insured has great relevance to some of the current proposals now being offered to "reduce the number" of uninsured Americans. Proposals for premium support (as through vouchers) or refundable tax credits would yield a very poor value in today's health care market. Even with generous premium support or tax credits, a person or family seeking insurance coverage in the individual market would still find it unaffordable, especially if there should be a preexisting condition. A recent analysis of the individual insurance market by the Kaiser Family Foundation showed a bleak picture of that market. For example, 35 percent of people applying for insurance were just turned down cold.[22]

Myth #10: Universal Coverage Will Overburden Our System

WE DON'T HAVE THE RESOURCES to handle the increased demand for services that would result from universal coverage. The assumption is that if we were to "open the floodgates," the system would be overwhelmed by the pent-up demands for health care from people who were formerly uninsured. In fact, this myth points out the woeful inadequacy of our current system for taking care of the uninsured. The myth also reveals two major faults of our present system: (1) the undersupply of primary care providers compared with the relative oversupply (there are exceptions) of specialists—a prime example of this is a report from the May 2005 AMA newsletter, which revealed that the number of third-year residents in internal medicine who intended to pursue a career in primary care fell from 54 percent in 1998 to an appalling 27 percent in 2003; and (2) the geographic maldistribution of our health care services. Both of these shortcomings are evidence of the market's failure to work for health care.

If the millions of Americans who delay care because they're afraid of the cost came in earlier, it would take stress *off* of the system. Clinicians all appreciate how much less time and effort it takes to care for people who are well compared to the time demands and resource-consuming hassles that accompany medical catastrophes. Yes, there would be a backlog of "catch-up" work that would need to be addressed. But the later we start to deal with the fruits of our neglect, the harder it will be to catch up. There's no doubt that the system needs to change. It must be more responsive to real health care needs, not just the whim of "the market." We have to make it more efficient. And in the reorganization of the system, first priority needs to go to patients and their needs.

Universal coverage should lead to the more appropriate use of emergency rooms (ERs) once people have improved access to primary care. ERs would be used for true emergencies, instead of the host of nonemergency cases that now clog their corridors. We'll have to find ingenious ways to meet an initial excess demand in a timely manner. We have a sufficient number of health care providers—even nurses, if we count all the nurses who now do administrative duties or who have left nursing out of frustration over adverse working conditions.

The possible solutions include: (1) more efficient use of primary care providers (with decreased administrative tasks, they should be able to do more patient care); (2) shifting of some specialist time into primary care; (3) increased use of mid-level clinicians, such as nurse practitioners and physician assistants; and (4) extra rewards for doing primary care in areas that are medically underserved. Eventually, when the "delayed care backlog" is caught up, the excess utilization should even out. The controversial issue of whether Americans are overutilizers of care will be discussed more fully in Chapter 2.

Myth #11: Costs of "Research and Development" Drive Our Higher Drug Prices

DRUG PRICES ARE HIGHER in the United States because our pharmaceutical industry spends billions of dollars on research and development. All the evidence shows this assertion to be a myth, a figment of creative accounting. The drug companies have the highest profit margin of all American corporations. Their profits as a percent of sales run about 19 percent, compared to a median of about 5 percent for all the Fortune 500 companies.[23] Data from the drug companies' annual reports show that they spend almost three times as much on marketing and administrative costs as they spend on research and development (R&D)[24]—a discrepancy totally ignored in a July 2002 HHS report linking innovation in drug development to the freedom from government controls.[25]

The drug companies claim that it costs them over $800 million (a recent number, it used to be only $500 million) to bring a new drug to market. This number is grossly exaggerated. Creative accounting—akin to the type used by Enron—has been used to inflate the true costs. They have included such items as "lost-opportunity costs" in doing their calculations. Other experts who have examined the data come up with much lower figures for R&D. Their estimates are closer to $100 million, a huge difference. *Public Citizen* put its estimate of the real number at $110 million (for 2000).[26]

Drug prices are much higher in America than in any other country—about 60 percent higher, on the average, than the prices in Canada and the United Kingdom. Our drug companies claim that the U.S. pharmaceutical industry carries the burden of doing R&D for the rest of the world. Yet the European countries

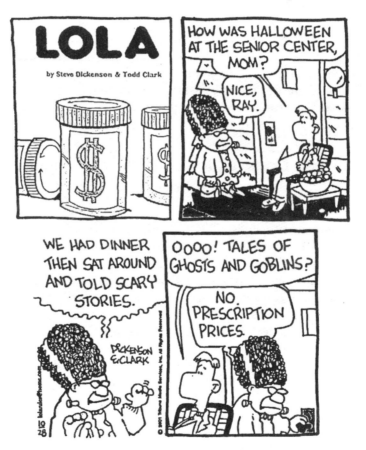

(combined) put out approximately the same number of new drugs a year as we do in America. And our drug industry's R&D gets huge taxpayer subsidies from government-supported drug research done by our National Institutes of Health and American universities.[27]

Our patent laws allow new drugs to become mini-monopolies, with "anything goes" pricing. And, with all of the new drugs produced in America, only a very small percentage are in fact innovative developments. Most are varieties of old drugs, like an extended-release product, developed to extend patent protections. Community needs are given a low priority. The reason drugs cost more in America than in any other country boils down to one simple factor: the pursuit of maximum profit. The pharmaceutical industry has taken every opportunity, used every ploy, to deceive the American people.

Some of the other questionable, and often illegal, ploys used by the pharmaceutical industry include:

- Manipulating patent law to keep cheaper generic products off the market (as with Taxol),[28] or paying off smaller pharmaceutical companies not to manufacture cheaper generic versions of their drugs, as has happened with BuSpar and Hytrin.[29]

- Giving kickbacks to physicians who overcharge Medicare for drugs. TAP Pharmaceuticals paid a record $875 million fine for abuses involving their prostate cancer drug Lupron.

- Price-fixing. In a case involving vitamins, several pharmaceutical companies paid a fine of more than $700 million.

- Paying off the "pharmaceutical benefit managers" who are supposed to save money for health care organizations by selecting cheaper drugs. They gave them bonuses for promoting drugs that were not always the most economical.[30]

- The systematic "bribing" of the medical profession and our legislators through an array of questionable but legal activities, from gifts and free lunches to campaign contributions.[31]

- The creation of so-called "Astroturf" grassroots support groups, like "Citizens for a Better Medicare," to give the impression there is popular support for or against a particular issue, such as a prescription benefit as an integral part of Medicare.

In its pursuit of profitability, the pharmaceutical industry is one of the most formidable obstacles to health care reform in America. Spending on their products has been increasing by 15 to 20 percent a year. With pharmaceutical costs about to surpass physician costs, only hospital costs are higher. The pharmaceutical industry enjoys enormous privileges in the form of generous tax benefits and patent protections. They operate without price controls, a unique circumstance among the developed nations of the world. They are performing a superb job in carrying out their mission to maximize stockholder profits, even if it means that millions of elderly Americans must choose between medicines or food.

Marcia Angell, the former editor of the *New England Journal of Medicine*, argues in an editorial that because of the pharmaceutical industry's large taxpayer subsidy, and "because it makes products of vital importance to the public health, it should be accountable not only to its shareholders, but also to society at large."[32]

Myth #12: We Can Get to Universal Coverage Through Incremental Changes

WE CAN GET TO UNIVERSAL COVERAGE through incremental or piecemeal changes. When the overly complex Clinton Plan died in 1994, efforts ceased for a comprehensive solution to help the uninsured. It seems that about every decade or so some momentum builds towards enacting universal coverage. In the past century, these efforts have routinely been beaten back each time—usually by a coalition of well-financed and politically influential interest groups. The traditional opponents of comprehensive change such as national health insurance have been the AMA, the insurance industry, the pharmaceutical industry, and certain other business interests. After the reform debacle of 1994, politicians looked at comprehensive change with the deference owed a third rail. Popular wisdom dictated that the only politically safe route to take in efforts at health care reform was the path of "incremental" change.

What have the incremental efforts of the past decade brought us? We've seen an increase of about 8 million in the number of the uninsured with nearly 3,200 a day being added to the roll. After a brief period of relative cost containment, thanks to the temporary effects of managed care and the denial of care to millions, we saw several years of double-digit health care inflation, and it continues to outstrip the growth of our economy by two to three times! And despite an ambitious (and, in some states, relatively successful) State Children's Health Insurance Program (SCHIP), the number of uninsured children remains only minimally reduced.

And now, with a seemingly reborn interest in increasing health insurance coverage, there is a plethora of ideas and proposals that have been accompanied by a lot of talk but so far not much action. They use the word "universal" fleetingly but really seem to mean "incremental." Foundations and the federal government (through HRSA) are paying millions of dollars to consultants and planners to come up with bold new ideas for providing health care coverage for more Americans. Many of the proposals, as noted above, are not really about "universal" coverage. Even in their broadest implementation, most of the plans leave millions of Americans uncovered. Instead of truly being bold, they defer to the fickle god of "political reality."

Reflecting our present quagmire of health insurance options, the new proposals postulate a complex and confusing array of approaches. Using the expansion of Medicaid and SCHIP as an initial step, they propose a mix of refundable tax credits, federal subsidies, health savings accounts, vouchers, employer-defined contributions, supplemental insurance policies to cover drugs or items that primary insurance doesn't cover, and buying cooperatives—among other ideas.

For my patients and millions of other Americans like them, the complexity of many of these proposals makes them pipe dreams. They are simply too complex and costly for the average near-poor family without health insurance, as well as for the growing millions who are inadequately insured. Each little part of these "incremental" or "piecemeal" approaches would likely help a limited number of people. But the added complexity will only serve to raise the overall administrative costs. And more people (perhaps different ones) will fall between the ever-enlarging cracks in the system. Meanwhile, the complexity enables the corporate groups with the smartest consultants and lawyers to continue to game the system.

In an essay looking at universal coverage in the United States from a historical perspective, Karen Davis, president of the Commonwealth Fund, remarks that "incremental changes that expand coverage but do not change the organization and delivery of services have fared better than more sweeping health care reform proposals that would have a substantial impact on the economic interests of health care providers and insurers."[33] Comprehensive change is difficult, yet "incremental" approaches have been slow and frustrating. Speaking of the uninsured in 1998, Drew Altman, president of the Kaiser Family Foundation, said, "We have been making some progress with the small incremental reforms, but it's like shoveling sand against the tide."

What about expansion of the federal programs, Medicare, Medicaid, and SCHIP? The Medicaid and/or SCHIP route has been the "incremental" path that most states have chosen to pursue. These approaches offer generous matching funds from Washington, up to 80 percent in the case of SCHIP. Some states, such as Rhode Island, have included people up to 400 percent of the poverty level in the programs. Several states are starting to cover parents of SCHIP beneficiaries. Yet most states have been much less generous. They see Medicaid and SCHIP, even with the federal match, as an increasingly onerous drain on their state budgets. Even the federal matching funds are beginning to dwindle. With recent legislation, billions of federal dollars are being slashed from the Medicaid program and with more and more people being considered eligible and the U.S. government facing a $9 trillion deficit, the whole system is unsustainable and heading for collapse.

States like Oregon and Minnesota have been innovative in their program design but, at least in the case of Oregon, the results have been far from adequate. The August 1, 2001, Portland *Oregonian* reported a study that showed 43 percent of the people covered by the Oregon Health Plan, the state's medical safety net for the poor, leave the plan within a year. They left largely because they earned just a little too much to qualify, but they still couldn't afford private insurance. A case example from our practice illustrates the dilemma:

> *Eighteen-year-old Mindy seriously injured her shoulder at work 10 months ago. She required surgery and Workmen's Compensation paid for it. Four months later, she reinjured the shoulder and was seen at the ER. The ER physician told her to follow up with a bone specialist, but she didn't since she couldn't afford it. Instead, she came to our health center 2 months later with a badly deformed shoulder. We determined that she would qualify for SCHIP, so we arranged an appointment with a bone specialist. Unfortunately, SCHIP expires at age 19 and she turned 19 just 2 days later, so she lost her insurance coverage and is once again unable to pay for care.*

Medicaid theoretically has an excellent benefit package, though it varies widely from state to state, as do the eligibility requirements. It also has nearly no co-pays, but as it exists today, Medicaid is far from ideal. It reimburses poorly. It's often difficult to find providers who will take patients with Medicaid, especially for dental services. Each state program is at the mercy of state budget-setters on a year-to-year basis. And Medicaid has a stigma attached to it, the aura of welfare. A recent study in the *American Journal of Public Health* on problems with access to dental care for Medicaid-insured children illustrates this phenomenon. Summarizing the results of that study:

> *"Negative experiences with the dental care system discouraged many caregivers . . . from obtaining dental services for their . . . children. . . . Caregivers who*

*successfully negotiated [the many logistic] barriers felt
that they encountered additional barriers in the dental
care setting, including long waiting times and judgmental,
disrespectful, and discriminatory behavior from staff
and providers because of their race and public assistance
status.*"[34]

Medicaid's worst problem is perhaps its impermanence for
individuals. Because of Medicaid's eligibility requirements,
many people have only transient coverage. They can get easily
dropped from the program. This fickle nature of Medicaid especially affects the working near-poor, many of whom are without
insurance today. Yet manipulating Medicaid and/or SCHIP, with
or without federal waivers, is by far the simplest means of doing
"incremental" change in a state. Arizona used the Medicaid
expansion tactic in 2000 by deciding to provide Medicaid coverage for all people up to 100 percent of poverty. However, with the
economic recession, all Medicaid approaches, including
Arizona's, are endangered.

In a recent article about Medicaid, Sara Rosenbaum explores
its precarious current situation.[35] Tight state budgets and the
newly available waivers threaten to trim benefits for people with
Medicaid. Only a short while ago, Medicaid and SCHIP were
"the low-lying fruit" for planners looking at ways to expand coverage. No more.

One peculiar aspect of Medicaid that has pretty much
escaped scrutiny is its relation to nursing homes. As the major
payer for nursing home services (an irrationality of its role—why
shouldn't Medicare be the payer?), Medicaid expenses for nursing homes have been fairly untouchable. Since nursing home
reimbursements represent about half of Medicaid costs (averag-
ing nearly $71,000 per nursing home resident per year), states are
fairly hamstrung when it comes to cutting services. It has become
a reverse "lifeboat" paradigm: dump the women and children
first. Meanwhile, the nursing homes are incredibly squeezed and
care is inadequate. A government study released in February
2002 reported that over 90 percent of U.S. nursing homes lacked
adequate staffing.[36] Registered nurse positions were found to be
staffed at barely over half the recommended level.

The Commonwealth Fund's 2000 proposal for (near) universal coverage—again, the play on words—envisages a great expansion of Medicaid to include all low-income people. And it puts high-risk people into Medicare. The healthy and relatively wealthy would be left for the private sector. It would be far from universal, do nothing to decrease administrative costs or complexity, and give a huge gift to the insurance industry. Moreover, it would further institutionalize a multitiered health care system in the United States.

As Uwe Reinhardt, the Princeton health economist, said about "incremental" reforms in 1999, "The problem lies in the self-destruct mechanism inherent in the very idea of incrementalism. Even Mother Teresa probably could not make incrementalism work any better. It has been thus and it always will be thus."[37]

We are seeing a variety of efforts toward incremental change today. Some, like myself, who advocate for comprehensive change, nonetheless pursue some of the incremental efforts *du jour,* such as follow-up care for women who are found to have breast cancer, because our patients are in need. Although they see the need, others have given up on trying to get comprehensive change. For them, incremental changes appear to be the only direction feasible in today's political climate. These well-intentioned people pursuing the route of noncomprehensive incremental change are pragmatists, as I am also on certain days. Many of them have become discouraged and have lost faith, at least temporarily.

The vested interests may have more cynical reasons for encouraging incremental change. They appreciate that such limited tweaking of the system will basically maintain the status quo and thereby assure the present balance of power and profits. The more cynical among them also may be encouraging the incremental path because it gives the appearance of doing *something* while avoiding the more fundamental questions. It's uncertain how long such stopgap measures such as discount coupons for drugs or reinsurance for inadequate insurance will forestall a real revolution in health care financing, a grassroots uprising that will eventually demand that health care be a right, and not a privilege, in the United States.

Are there incremental-type changes that can lead to a just system of universal coverage? Probably yes. The types of progressive or "sequential" incremental change that could lead to universal coverage could be measures that are all-inclusive of a specific age group of our population. For example, we could put all children, or all people aged 55 to 64, in an expanded Medicare as a first step. Similarly, a state-by-state strategy (as a first step) could also work as it did in Canada, but it would be much more difficult because of the legal hurdles that would have to be overcome. At least these kinds of approaches would obviate the gaming of the system that excludes the sick and the poor.

Then there is the incremental approach proposed in April 2002 by the American College of Physicians–American Society of Internal Medicine. It meets the criterion of progressively reaching the goal of universal coverage (everyone included). They outline how universal coverage could be reached in stages over 7 years. But the proposal's framework is built upon expansion of Medicaid and SCHIP with the addition of premium support. Although they admit they are dealing exclusively with the issue of "coverage," they are skirting the issue of affordability. Instead of addressing the failures, inefficiencies, and inequities of our current fragmented system, they are taking the approach of "throwing money at the system"—feeding the monster. As of the time of this second edition, it has been nearly 5 years since the "incremental" proposal paper brought forth by the ACP was published. It is interesting to note that many of the ideas put forward have actually been adopted (or seriously considered) and that the current health care policies of the Bush administration seem to follow their philosophy. Sadly, yet predictably, we are no better off. The supposed monies available for the government "safety net" are actually dwindling, health care inflation continues to outpace the country's economic growth by a factor of 3, and the number of uninsured and poorly insured continues to grow and is quickly becoming pervasive in mainstream middle-class America.

Although it's uncertain how long the economy will continue to suffer, the current worsening economic situation bodes poorly for the success of incremental approaches. With increasing unemployment, a growing number of uninsured, rapidly rising health care costs, and a diminishing ability to fund government-financed "safety-net" programs like Medicaid, we need a more comprehensive solution. As David Broder said in an op-ed piece in the *Washington Post*, "It is . . . clear that tinkering around the edges cannot, for long, withstand the adverse trends that are at work, let alone reverse them."[38]

Myth #13: Americans Won't Accept Single-Payer Universal Coverage

AMERICANS WILL NEVER ACCEPT a single-payer system. This myth, which will be explored in more detail in Chapters 14 and 15, is a particularly critical point for the vested interests. The special-interest groups that promote this myth take every opportunity to exclude single-payer advocates from discussions of health care reform. They assert that we must have a "pluralistic" approach to health care reform, thereby assuring their hegemony. The American people, who have been exposed only to the rhetoric of the vested interests, have not had the opportunity to form any thoughtful consensus on the single-payer approach. The merchants of misinformation and myth have been successful at hawking a line of philosophic incompatibility to discredit the single-payer approach—"we hate government, we don't want socialized medicine."

Columnist Molly Ivins noted: "Every time we start to get serious about reform, the right wing starts screaming, 'Socialized medicine, socialized medicine.' And then we're all supposed to run screaming with horror."[39] Ivins goes on to endorse the type of solution that every other industrialized country has embraced: "Universal health insurance, a single-payer system." Single payer is not "socialized medicine," nor does it need to be "big government."

Unfortunately, the term "single payer" is oversimplified. Even advocates for universal coverage disagree on the use of the term. But in general, "single payer" identifies an approach based on "one risk pool" with everyone included, like national health insurance. A summary of the principles that comprise the "single-payer" with "one risk pool" type of solution is found at the end of the Introduction to this book.

Can you imagine what a national health insurance system with group (meaning, every American) clout could do in negotiating discounts in drug prices? If I were the pharmaceutical industry, I'd worry—and they do. Their $38 billion in profits in 2000 could be cut in half, although there are reasonable theories that argue that increased sales under a program of national health insurance would offset the losses from lower prices. It's not hard to wonder why they spend so many millions on lobbying, campaign contributions, and expensive advertising campaigns. As for the health insurance industry, they would be fighting for their very existence.

How about the AMA? As a physician, I'm ashamed of them. They've forgotten the primary mission of physicians as caregivers. As an organization, the AMA has lost touch with reality. They have little appreciation for what it means to be uninsured. Nor do they know how little it really matters to be able to exercise "personal responsibility" in the chaotic, fragmented, and illogical health care environment that exists in America today.

Americans overwhelmingly support universal coverage, yet they are largely doubtful that we can accomplish the goal. Their doubt is the result of a purposeful campaign of misinformation and disinformation to "keep America clueless." The mythology works to create the sense that universal coverage with a single-payer-type system is a pipe dream, not to be considered seriously. For the moment, it's politically difficult to promote the single-payer approach, like Medicare for All or national health insurance. But the winds of politics can change in the blink of an eye.

Though economic conditions in America can change quickly, the near future appears to be bringing deterioration in the status of both the uninsured and the insured. America is facing the danger of a "health care meltdown" that will threaten the well-being of middle-class America. Many more middle-class Americans will be hurting. Grassroots indignation and unrest could ensue, with a demand for real change in how we finance health care in this country. In 2000, a ballot initiative for single-payer-type universal coverage just barely missed passage (48 percent to 52 percent) in Massachusetts.

How long can the special interests maintain the myths? More importantly, how much longer will the American people tolerate having their own health care needs kept subservient to the self-serving goals of the special-interest groups? Only as long as the American people can be kept clueless.

Unfortunately, the myths have helped to maintain and nurture the "monster" that our American health care system has become. The following two chapters explore this "monster."

Summary of Key Points

- The American people have been led to believe a series of myths about our health care system, myths that impede change.

- "The market" has been a failure for health care in America. Health care is not a commodity like fast food or automobiles.

- For health care, the public sector in fact has a much lower overhead than the private sector.

- There is a better way: universal coverage with "one risk pool."

- Health care for all is affordable, but will require basic reforms of our current crazy, dysfunctional system.

- Incremental approaches have not led to significant change in our system but have only delayed the implementation of real change.

- "One risk pool" with everybody in—and nobody out—is *not* socialized medicine.

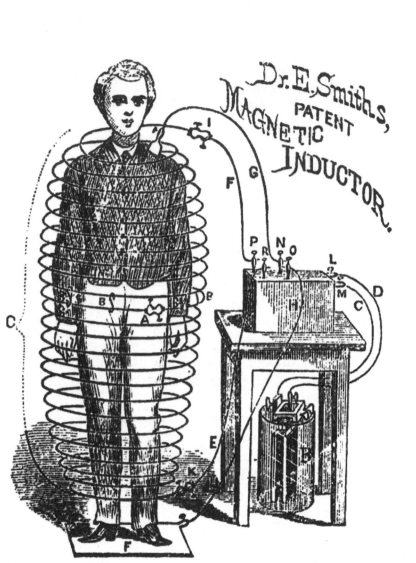

Dr. E. Smith's, PATENT MAGNETIC INDUCTOR.

If not called for in 10 days P. M. return to
Dr. E. SMITH, Normal, Ills.

Chapter 2

America's Health Care:
The Monster We Have Created

". . . As soon as I started to learn about health care and health insurance, I was so struck by the craziness of the system and how unjust it is and how it makes no sense."
—Health policy expert Rima Cohen[1]

The 72-year-old woman was overweight and had diabetes. She also had a stuffy nose and railroad insurance that covered the cost of prescriptions not covered by Medicare. Instead of buying an inexpensive over-the-counter medication, she asked that I prescribe a $90 a month non-sedating kind of antihistamine. "My insurance pays for it," she said. "I don't care what it costs."

Another woman, 64 years old, has diabetes and high blood pressure. She misses her appointments and tells me that she takes her medicines only two or three times a week because, "Doc, that's all I can afford." Her blood sugar is 300 (normal being about 100) and her blood pressure 160/110 (normal being less than 140/90).

QUITE POSSIBLY, FRANZ KAFKA and Dr. Frankenstein were collaborators in the design of our American health care system, and they carried out their work with grant funding from the Alfred Hitchcock Foundation. Or so it seems. The United States has always had an aversion to health planning ("socialism!"), but our love of laissez-faire "free-market" principles has helped create a "monster" of a health care system, or more correctly stated, nonsystem. And as we struggle with the difficulty of implementing change in America, we are seeing our already deficient health system get even worse. Perhaps Mr. Kafka has returned as the CEO of an HMO.

"My insurance covers MRIs, doc. So I'd like to have one." How often have we physicians heard this request, or others like it for a variety of tests, procedures, or referrals? "I've got a pain in my knee. I need a referral to a bone doctor." I recently saw a 60-year-old man with heart disease who saw an ad for the blood thinner Plavix on TV. He asked me to prescribe it for him (at $110 a month) instead of the daily aspirin he was taking—even though he wouldn't quit smoking. These requests often come without any discussion. I've had patients (insured, of course) request total body CAT scans to help tell them why they have some vague aches and pains—again, even before discussing the symptoms. Meanwhile, those very tests are being marketed to the public— no doctor's referral necessary.

On the other hand, the uninsured patients want as little done as possible. "Please, doc, no lab tests today. I can't afford them." But it's amazing what "catch-up" medical work gets done when someone gets health insurance or turns 65 and qualifies for Medicare. Suddenly the gallbladder that's been acting up off and on for 8 years is taken out, the diagnostic tests for angina are done. Perhaps most frustrating for me as a physician are the chronic disease patients who won't return for needed follow-ups because they can't afford the visits. These are the people with poorly controlled hypertension, diabetes, or heart disease, who "live with" their ailments. Even at our community health center, which has a (now) $10 "nominal" fee for a visit, many won't come back until they're out of medications—or worse.

There's a disconnect here. Although these are a few simple examples of the paradoxes and inequities in our system, health care in America, as it has evolved in a haphazard way, is really extremely complicated and full of contradictions, inefficiencies, and chaos. A "health care hodgepodge," as the *Des Moines Register* editorial board termed it in an editorial piece.[2] If we were to look at our system from the outside, we could easily conclude that, given our generous resources as the richest country in the world, we couldn't have designed a more dysfunctional system if we had tried.

In his recent book, *As Sick as It Gets*,[3] Rudy Mueller, MD, describes in minute and excruciating detail just how frightful our system has become. He relates how it affects people's daily lives and robs them not only of their money, but also of their dignity. I see the horrors of our nonsystem every day in my own community health center practice. The irrationality, the inhumanity, the greed, the inequity, and even the cruelty are incomprehensible for a nation that wants to believe "we have the best health care system in the world."

It's not that millions of American health care workers, from receptionists to physicians, are not trying to do their best to serve patients with diligence and compassion. I see many good-faith efforts to help people every day. But our broken system puts unnecessary (and often senseless) obstacles in the way of people getting the health care they need. And the self-destructiveness of the system has only accelerated in the past two decades with the transformation of American health care from what was primarily a caring endeavor to a commercial enterprise. Kathleen O'Connor, in her book *The Buck Stops Nowhere*,[4] demonstrates the perversion of our system in her first chapter on "healthcare's battlefield." She devotes 36 pages of that chapter to the games of financing and "the market" and less than two pages to "the patient." Our priorities have been turned upside down.

We've created a huge monster. We continue to nourish the monster because powerful financial interest groups, like the pharmaceutical industry, the insurance companies, large employers, and some elements of the medical establishment, know that any real solution could threaten their bottom lines. So they have helped to create a mythology to plant the doubt that Americans who are already insured might lose something if there were to be any real changes.

Thus, we see a series of proposals to "tweak the monster" and make it more complicated and incomprehensible—all to delay the inevitable (real change). And to heck with the patients. They are being enticed to pay more and more of the costs while being lulled to complacency by flowery phraseology such as "more choice," "consumer-directed care," or "health savings accounts." The monster continues to grow, and as it grows, it devours our resources and squelches any good intentions. The monster has many dimensions.

Managed Care vs. Managed Cost: "Crazy Making"

MUCH HAS BEEN WRITTEN and debated on the experience with "managed care" in America, a uniquely American experience in "crazy making," especially for *insured* Americans. The response of Americans to a movie like "John Q," which portrays how the managed-care industry "jerks people around" and denies needed care, demonstrates how much health insurers have come to be reviled by the American public—perhaps second only to the tobacco industry.

Managed care itself is basically a sound concept. The alternative, "unmanaged care"—care delivered without regard to scientific evidence, cost, or relevance to the individual or society—is clearly inappropriate. The current trend towards rational "disease management" is a positive aspect of managed care. America's prime example of the old style of managed care, Kaiser Permanente, a not-for-profit group health plan, had, and still has, many favorable qualities. Responding to a recent flawed analysis in the *British Medical Journal*,[5] which compared California's Kaiser Permanente to Britain's National Health System (NHS), health policy expert Kevin Grumbach remarked that, "Within the disorganized and inefficient context of the overall U.S. health care system, Kaiser does stand out as an admirable model of health care integration . . . ."[6]

But managed care in America has gone astray. Its original purpose, as with the old Kaiser model, was to coordinate and improve patient care. However, when the concept was applied to eliminating waste and inefficiencies in the health care system, not a bad end in itself, the whole emphasis changed to "managed cost." The patient focus was lost and became a secondary goal.

The result has been more "mangled cared" than "managed care." "The market" and economic interests became the driving force for health care in America. As a local employer explained to me, he had three motivations for embracing managed care: "Cost, cost, and cost." As a result, the insured in America have been "jerked around"—and will continue to be "jerked around"—by insurers and employers if we continue in the direction we appear to be headed.

Movies like "John Q" and the Showtime movie released in May 2002, "Damaged Care," touch a raw nerve with the American public. "Damaged Care" tells the true story of Linda Peeno, MD, who, as medical director of Humana, was forced to deny care systematically so that profits could be maximized for the corporation. Most people, however, have little appreciation for the abuses of "managed cost" until they (or one of their family members) have a serious illness and a hands-on encounter with the managed-care industry. Many Americans come away from the experience with a total disbelief of just how crazy—and uncaring—our system has become. And as our system heads towards "meltdown," the situation will only get worse, especially for middle-class Americans.

Unrealistic Expectations

FROM "MARCUS WELBY," TO "ER," to media splashes about technological advances such as mechanical hearts and limb replacements, even to the "direct-to-consumer" ads pushing cures for toenail fungus or seasonal allergies, the American public has been led to expect wonders from our health care system. The smiling, athletic people in the HMO ads don't expect to have their claims denied when they show up in the ER without preauthorization. And people expecting to spend an hour discussing their health care concerns with Dr. Welby, Jr., don't realize that Doc Welby is expected to see 28 patients a day.

In all fairness, many of the expectations have the potential to be real, at least technologically. Our technology is wonderful. There have been especially great advances in pharmacology. For example, new drugs have nearly eliminated bleeding stomach ulcers and the need for ulcer surgery. The "statin" drugs provide great promise to prevent heart attacks and strokes. New antidepressants and antipsychotics have provided huge advances in the treatment of mental illness. Many of these advances have led to a substantial decrease in the need for hospitalization.

Meanwhile, there have been equally huge leaps forward in such areas as joint replacements, microsurgical techniques, and diagnostic testing, offering an improved state of well-being for many. Surgical procedures that used to require long hospitalizations are now done in day surgery with much less discomfort and trauma for the patient. Future developments in areas such as gene therapy and even greater miniaturization will create a whole new array of possibilities; for example, curing diabetes or cancer, or even halting the aging process.

But these expectations have been largely divorced from realistic cost factors or affordability. And prevention has taken a distant back seat to expensive and media-hyped interventions aimed at curing illness or fixing injury. Americans, like our health care industry, think short term. The new technologies are at times amazing and, of course, usually very expensive. But, after all, if it were available, who wouldn't want the "very best" treatment, especially if it were covered by insurance? If your child were ill, wouldn't you want the treatment with the highest chance of success, even if it cost a bundle?

Pharmaceutical industry dollars and the media attention given to medical and technological advances have changed the culture of how Americans look at health care. Americans have come to "expect the world." Of course, the argument could be made that people *should* be able to "expect the world" even though that might involve forgoing something else or resorting to statewide bake sales to pay the bill. The message from the sellers of health care, and the way physicians used to be taught to practice, has clearly been to ignore cost and do the "very best," though it hasn't always been clear that the "very best" is really best. Although the managed-cost gurus have tried to modify the message, physicians' training (at least in the old days) never talked about "Option #2—use in case of uninsurance."

Interestingly enough, there are rifts among the major health care players on this issue of pursuing the "very best" for patients. The pharmaceutical industry and medical specialists push their expensive and often, but not always, more efficacious options. But the insurance industry and managed-care organizations fight to control costs. So the two sides are sometimes at loggerheads, as with the issue of converting certain expensive antihistamines from prescription-only to over-the-counter (OTC) status. Such a change would help insurers, who don't normally pay for OTC drugs. But it would hurt the pharmaceutical companies because people would balk at paying $80 a month out of pocket for a drug when they could buy an almost equivalent product for a few dollars.

Crazy pricing is a major factor in driving up costs. Historically, providers were able to collect whatever they charged, and this "history" has served to perpetuate a system with excessively high price tags, most notably for specialist care and "procedures." "Thinking" clinicians (that is, clinicians who use cognitive approaches versus procedural interventions) might get reimbursed $35 for talking to a patient for half an hour about multiple medical problems, but pass a tube to someone's stomach (it can be done in 10 minutes) and the payment can be $900. Illogical, but that's our system. Mostly, we've saddled the system with overpayments, but there are also underpayments, as made to clinicians who care for Medicaid and some HMO or Medicare patients. Many physicians now refuse to take on patients with Medicaid and/or Medicare if they have enough full-paying patients. Crazy pricing has been particularly harmful for the uninsured and the underinsured. They are increasingly being forced to choose "Option #2" or "Option #3" (no care).

Instead of "great expectations," a large number of Americans must settle for "small expectations," like a woman we recently saw with a 10-inch mass in her abdomen. She's unable to find a surgeon to take out her tumor because she can't afford $1,900 up front. After all, that's the way "the market" works. And that's a major reason why there is a fundamental disconnect between "the market" and health care in America.

Ignorance of the Costs

HEALTH ECONOMIST UWE REINHARDT has politely described the way we price health care in America as "one of the most opaque sectors in the economy."[7] He adds, "Many folks must prefer it that way, or it would not be so." Only recently have there been some efforts to educate caregivers about costs. But there appears to be almost no effort yet to educate patients on this critical issue—thus, keeping the demand unabated for, say, expensive drugs. I don't see prices advertised in the glitzy ads for Sporanox, Nexium, or Claritin. It doesn't state in the direct-to-consumer ads that the treatment for toenail fungus costs $800 per course of therapy, or that the "purple pill" for heartburn will cost $120 a month as opposed to Zantac, which can work just as well for a fraction of the cost. It's to the advantage of the pharmaceutical companies for patients to have little idea what their drugs cost. With inpatient care, the patient may never even see the hospital bill if it's paid for by private insurance. Medicare beneficiaries who do see the bottom line of their bill are blown away by the amount.

Physicians used to be taught to forget the cost. The drug reps never used to discuss cost, and now they usually bring it up when they're trying to show how much cheaper their product is compared to their competitors' (for example, only $110 a month versus $130). As for diagnostic tests, we physicians hardly ever think of their cost. We order them and expect the patient to get what we ordered. Also unaware of the costs, the patient usually complies. Both the physician and the patient are then surprised when (and if) they find out that the prenatal ultrasound cost $600 or the echocardiogram cost $1,000.

Squeezed by economic pressures, hospitals have started to try to educate their doctors on the relative costs of the drugs they prescribe in the hospital, especially since Medicare now gives a fixed diagnosis-related reimbursement for each hospital patient. And managed-care plans have been highly motivated to try to educate their physicians on drug costs. They have created drug formularies, which make sense in theory, but are based mostly on cost, not efficacy. The formularies often complicate matters for the patient, who may be forced to switch drugs and then suffer unfortunate side effects.

We could do much more to lower costs, such as practicing scientifically based medicine, but it's like combating an epidemic. There is such a strong incentive, as with the pharmaceutical industry and surgical subspecialists, to keep prices—and profits or incomes—high. It will likely require a major change in how we organize health care in America to effect any meaningful change. If we were really to practice scientifically based medicine, the cost savings would be great. We order and do so many unnecessary tests and procedures, and our prescribing patterns are illogical and expensive.

Switching from the individual patient to the macroeconomic scale, ignorance of true costs has created major opportunities for maximizing profits. The insurance companies benefit greatly from playing the "ignorance game," as described in a Web article entitled "What your health insurer doesn't want you to know."[8] Manipulation of the system, using its complexity and its financial "opacity," has become the norm for health care in America. Arrangements that unnecessarily increase the cost of health care—beyond administrative costs—are being brought to light. Examples: the high added costs of commissions for insurance brokers; inflated drug costs for products supplied by "pharmaceutical benefit managers"; and, now, questionable practices by the middlemen who do the group purchasing of medical supplies for hospitals.

As described in an article in *The New York Times*,[9] two private groups (Premier and Novation), acting as middlemen for about half of America's not-for-profit hospitals, may have been compromising their mission to find the best supplies for hospitals at the lowest prices. It appears that the two buying groups, with purchases of $34 billion in 2001, "are financed not by the hospitals that buy the products but by the companies that sell them." The middlemen have financial ties to medical supply companies that are "both extensive and highly unusual." Buying groups are, in effect, getting paid to buy certain products. The situation illustrates how "the market" in health care has encouraged the development of oligopolies with a concomitant abuse of power.

It also shows how an industry managed to escape regulatory over-sight, as with Enron, by convincing Congress to exempt them from rules such as the federal anti-kickback laws.

The Paperwork Nightmare

THERE HAS BEEN A QUANTUM LEAP in the past 10 to 15 years in the amount of paperwork required to carry out the daily tasks of health care. Paralleling this growth in paperwork has been a vast expansion in the number of people required to administer our system (see the graph showing the comparative growth of physi-cians and administrators over the past 30 years).

Growth of Physicians and Administrators, 1970-1998

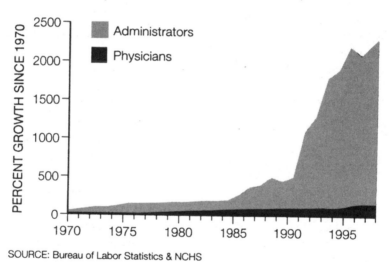

SOURCE: Bureau of Labor Statistics & NCHS

Reprinted with permission.

The fragmentation of insurance coverage, and the accompa-nying need for establishing eligibility for the various insurance programs, has greatly increased administrative costs and hassles. With respect to eligibility, health policy expert Sherry Glied points out that, "Universal coverage would readily solve all of the problems [with eligibility determination], as would a health insurance system that enrolled everyone automatically and then determined appropriate financing sources."[10] In other words, a single risk pool would simplify our system and require much less paperwork. The more recent increase in paperwork, which claims more and more of providers' time, has come both from the demands of managed-care organizations and from government efforts to stem fraud and abuse.

Some of the most onerous paperwork, sad to say, may be for Medicare, although not so much in the office setting. I pity the poor home health and nursing home workers who must spend three-quarters of their time writing notes about each patient. They cram endless handwritten notes into tiny writing so that the required information fits in the spaces provided. They can't possibly have much time left to care for the patients. Similarly, RNs in hospitals are consumed with filling out forms or completing notes. That's one of the prime reasons why nursing has lost its desirability as a profession. The situation cries out for improvement and simplification.

There's a story about nurses in hospitals being told by supervisors to avoid eye contact with patients when they go into the rooms. If they don't make eye contact, they will spend less time talking to the patient and, presumably, will have more time for their administrative chores.

The Medicare forms for durable medical equipment are complex, often incomprehensible, and take lengthy efforts to complete. If I could think of the number-one reason I would consider quitting the practice of medicine, it would be these forms. For hospitals, Medicare requirements are a burden, requiring extra staff and resources—resources that are diverted from patient care. But the managed-care companies have also done a good job of creating at least an equal burden of tedious paperwork for hospitals and other providers. Case in point: there's a story about Michael Dukakis visiting a large hospital in Vancouver, B.C., and asking to see its administrative wing. When he was shown two small rooms and told that was the entire billing department, he was flabbergasted. There are some things we could learn from Canada, even if the AMA and our pharmaceutical industry tell us their system is falling apart.

The type of administrative hassle that most rankles physicians involves not just paperwork but sometimes lengthy phone conversations required from managed-care organizations to obtain approval for patient referrals and/or diagnostic testing. Again, resources and time are diverted from patient care under the guise of controlling costs—costs that are then shifted to pay for administrative personnel. "Cost-shifting" used to mean using the receipts from private and government insurance to pay for indigent care. But our new definition of cost-shifting is taking resources from patient care to use for administration, profits, consultants, and, yes, paperwork.

Fraud and Abuse

THERE HAVE ALWAYS BEEN paperwork requirements in health care, and physicians have always complained about them: chart work, operative notes, transfer notes, and completing medical records in general. But the new brand of paperwork that has come about with managed care and anti-fraud efforts has added a whole new dimension, including new armies of bureaucratic personnel, to the paperwork nightmare.

In the private sector, the fragmentation of our system and the bureaucratic demands of managed care have driven the explosion of paperwork. A recent study of 2,277 people in the Seattle health insurance market found that they were covered by 755 different health insurance policies and 189 different health care plans.[11] But for the government programs, Medicare and Medicaid, a different cause is driving the paperwork monster. That cause pretty much boils down to an attempt to control fraud and abuse. Many players in American health care, following the gods of the entrepreneurial spirit, became a bit too zealous in the way they were gaming the system. Some of the "abuse" was out-and-out criminal fraud, perpetuated by people outside the system. The latter group found it easy, especially with the opportunities presented by electronic billing, to rob big bucks. When HCFA admitted that it had paid out $23 billion too much through fraudulent or inflated Medicare billings in 1998, people seemed to blame Medicare. But it wasn't Medicare that did the billings. It was the providers or crooks who submitted the inflated or fraudulent charges.

HCA/Columbia, the nation's largest for-profit hospital chain, systematically overcoded diagnoses to bilk Medicare. This was but one of their questionable practices to maximize their billings. They paid a "first installment" fine of $740 million to Medicare as part of a settlement. Even Illinois Blue Cross paid a fine of $140 million for ripping off Medicare. Nursing homes and a large number of bandit or fly-by-night home health agencies figured out ways to maximize charges, even for services not delivered.

Mental health has proven to be a prime profit center (through fraud) for both corporations that have mental health facilities and individuals who run "shelter homes." Some psychiatric hospitals were keeping patients for just as long as their insurance paid the bill, with little regard for the need. Tenet paid a $300 million fine for that practice. A series of articles in *The New York Times* has highlighted the abusive practices in the group shelter homes that house many of the mentally ill in New York City. Greed appears to be the driving motivation in their care. Many of the patients were subjected to assembly line-type surgeries, like prostate resections and cataract repairs, often with questionable indications. The profit motivation may have led to collusion between the shelter homes and greedy surgeons, who were able to bill Medicare or Medicaid for the procedures whether they were needed or not. The federal programs have also been systematically overbilled by diagnostic laboratories, which paid fines in the hundreds of millions of dollars and then kept on operating.

In the field of "durable medical equipment," the situation is wild. I recently got a card from a supplier outlining exactly what I needed to provide in the form of paperwork so that a fully ambulatory patient could get a motorized wheelchair. There was no indication of cost, and I suspect it would have been close to $5,000. The item, moreover, was unnecessary. The patient walked out of my office with relative ease. The markups on these items are incredible. Another one of my elderly patients, who had been hospitalized a few months earlier, had been discharged from the hospital with an oxygen concentrator for which Medicare was being billed $472 a month. At that price, she had assumed she was buying the machine (not so). She rarely used it. She informed me (I was totally unaware) that the renting company would not stop billing Medicare until I wrote an order to discontinue the machine.

Our system has also spawned a certain degree of patient fraud and abuse, though, dollar-wise, it is of a much lower order of magnitude compared to corporate stealing. The diversion and misuse of prescriptions, often related to substance abuse, has been a problem, especially with Medicaid. As a result, there has been a need for a growing bureaucracy to respond to the entrepreneurial efforts of some individuals.

Malcolm Sparrow, in his book, *License to Steal*,[12] goes into carefully documented detail to describe the extent to which fraud has undermined our American health care system. I get angry when I think of the care that my patients have effectively been denied because so much money has been diverted to what amounts to banditry, mostly of the corporate variety. The resultant mushrooming of administrative requirements adds insult to injury.

The Paperwork Could Get Worse

UNFORTUNATELY, THE PAPERWORK MONSTER could very easily get even worse in the near future. There are some experts who, in the belief that a single-payer government-directed solution is politically impossible, advocate for making the system *more* complex. They feel that it will take a greater degree of complexity to get more Americans insured. The types of solutions being suggested include vouchers, refundable tax credits, and employer-defined contributions. These all would: (1) increase the already ridiculous level of complexity in our health care financing system (thus increasing administrative costs and inequities); and (2) make health care even more unaffordable for low-income people.

Part of the solution to our present and future administrative and paperwork mess could come from improved electronic information systems. They have the potential to make the health care system more efficient and accountable as opposed to creating opportunities for stealing. Computer networks, electronic medical records, and the Internet all have great promise as tools to help improve our system. They could be especially effective in the dissemination of information and in the improvement of quality.

In practice, however, the information age is barely beyond its infancy in its day-to-day application to the practice of medicine. I'm not sure the patient visit aspect of health care will ever become as fully electronic as the financial side has become. And probably it shouldn't, despite the efforts of Newt Gingrich and some corporations to digitalize medicine (for example, the "Leapfrog Group") in the name of preventing errors.

Underutilization/Overutilization: (1) The "Underutilizers"

IT SEEMS ODD THAT knowledgeable people in the field of health care can argue over whether America's system suffers from too much underutilization or too much overutilization. There's no doubt that our schizophrenic health care system has both. And both have played an important role in the failure of our system to meet the needs of our nation. We have created a system with the wrong incentives.

In my practice I largely see a bias toward underutilization since nearly all of my patients are either uninsured or under-insured. Most of my Medicare patients qualify for the latter, as they are predominantly low-income seniors who have a difficult time paying for their medications, even with our help. Ironically, our safety-net clinics now see a growing number of people who have insurance. They come to us because they can't afford their deductibles and co-pays—or when they have been turned away elsewhere because their insurance has too many exceptions or limiting conditions. One evening I took care of a young woman who came to our clinic because she didn't have enough cash to pay for a visit elsewhere. Her plan required substantial co-payments for visits and full cash payment for prescriptions with reimbursement later. I had to be sure to prescribe inexpensive medications.

Because of the lack of insurance, as well as the barriers created by unaffordable deductibles and co-payments, people delay care until they're really sick. By and large, they have too much pride to ask for handouts from friends or family to cover the costs of care. So they often wait until they're *really* sick, like the 24-year-old woman who, fearful of the cost, waited several days to come to our clinic and then died the following day from a bacterial infection of her heart.

People with chronic diseases don't return for follow-up visits when they should. They ration their medicines, take a pill every other day when they're supposed to take it daily, or just quit the medicines altogether "because they feel okay." They don't like being badgered for payment, even for the co-pays they can't afford, so they sometimes return a year or two later, when they can no longer get their medications refilled. Some may have run out of their drugs a few months earlier, and they come in with very high blood sugars or elevated blood pressures. When they have catastrophes, like a heart attack, a stroke, or sudden blindness from a bleed in their eye, they're more expensive to treat and, of course, their suffering is greater.

Underutilization by Medicare beneficiaries is a phenomenon I see on an almost daily basis. With the changing economics of health care, Medicare has become a form of *under*insurance. When Medicare began in 1965, there were few expensive drugs. A study published in *JAMA* in 2000 by the RAND group on the utilization of services in Medicare fee-for-service (period 1994-1996) showed widespread underutilization of services deemed "necessary." This discrepancy was especially notable among black beneficiaries and in low-income areas. [13]

Underutilization is likely to become even more widespread in the near future as the cost of care rises and as employers increasingly shift more of the costs to employees. With a rising rate of unemployment, employers will feel less pressure to be generous with health care benefits. Employers are working with insurance companies to develop "defined-contribution" or "employee-driven" health care plans that give the appearance that they offer "more choice." But in fact, as with health savings accounts, for low-income Americans, as opposed to high-income people, these plans will only increase inequities in our health care system. Low-income people will pick the least expensive plans with the highest deductibles and co-pays because that will be all they can afford. And they will delay needed care. They will underutilize.

The strategy to increase deductibles and co-pays is based on the theory that these higher payments will discourage unnecessary use of services. But insurers and employers can't possibly *not* realize that these increased costs will also discourage the use of *necessary* care, most notably for lower-income people who are truly sick.

In the more global picture, underutilization is a major reason, if not *the* major reason, for our country's poor performance on the major health indicators vis-à-vis the other developed countries.

Critics have blamed our poor performance on poor folks who don't comply with their care. Well, of course, those poor folks, especially those from minority ethnic groups, don't comply. The system wasn't designed for them and their chaotic lives. That's the major reason for the existence of our "safety-net" clinics: the community health centers, the county hospitals, and the "health care for the homeless" programs.

But when we admonish these people for not complying, we're blaming the victims. We've created a health care system that creates barriers to their access to care. It's low-income people who go without the care, who raise our infant mortality rate and lower our life expectancy rate. They underutilize mostly because they can't afford it. Their resulting poor health creates a vicious cycle of poverty and, in the long run, affects our economic status—and our dignity—as a nation.

(2) The "Overutilizers"

THE CONTRASTING PHENOMENON, the overutilization of health care services, drains our system's resources while providing minimal added benefit—or even leading to harm. Overutilization, or even "alleged" overutilizaton, real or not real, has pushed insurers to increase deductibles and co-pays. Although lofty expectations from consumers do have a role in causing our system to be so expensive, the insane pricing of American health care is much more to blame. In allowing prices to evolve in such an irrational and counterproductive manner (where quality and reason have been eclipsed by the entrepreneurial spirit), "the market" has done a disservice to America's health care system and to the millions of Americans who must beg for care or do without. Then add to the inflated pricing the health care industry's lavish advertising campaigns and the media's hype on new technologies, and we have a formula for the hyperutilization of expensive services.

What about "entitlement chutzpah," the rationale behind the alleged overutilization and abuse of the system carried out by people who show up at ungodly hours at the ER? The people who demand care for trivial problems because they have Medicaid, and that covers all the charges, so why should they care? So goes the refrain from the docs who complain. I suspect that the people (docs and others) who gripe about Medicaid "abusers" are somewhat less upset by the "abuses" of people who have private insurance or adequate cash in hand. Prejudice against Medicaid recipients has likely become worse as people with commercial insurance have found themselves increasingly affected by higher out-of-pocket expenses. The Medicaid package is much more comprehensive and consumer-friendly than private insurance, and, therefore, it is often resented by people who must suffer high deductibles and co-pays. In Idaho, legislators cynically refer to Medicaid as "the gold card." The elements of class and racial discrimination also are a factor in the anti-entitlement sentiment so prevalent among many conservatives in America. The bias against minorities, even when they're insured, was documented in a recent study.

Yet, overutilization by poor people of color, or poor whites from Appalachia, with entitlements (Medicaid) constitutes only a minimal portion of the unnecessarily high spending of our health care system. All the evidence shows that poor people, even those with Medicaid, get fewer services, especially expensive services like cardiac catheterization, than middle-class people. The uninsured only use about 60 percent of the services used by the insured. It's more the high expectations of middle-class America, along with the willingness of providers to satisfy those expectations, that has led to the costly overutilization of expensive services. The word "expensive" is key. In Japan, with universal coverage and an average of 16 patient visits a year compared to about 6 in the United States,[14] they spend less than half of what we spend on health care despite the apparent gross overutilization.

Our American health care "monster" has created a situation where market hype has combined with (and helped create) inflated consumer expectations. The result has been a series of bizarre consequences, including inappropriate overutilization, as opposed to inappropriate underutilization by those who lack easy access. Unfortunately, as a result of perverse incentives, those least able to participate in the system have been penalized most. Not only do the patients come last in American health care today, but they also are blamed for the system's shortcomings.

How our system has evolved to create a litany of perverse incentives is further elaborated in the next chapter.

Summary of Key Points

- The American health care system is a hodge-podge, a complex nightmare that wastes billions that could be spent on needed health care.

- The health care and insurance pricing system is incredibly "opaque" and encourages waste, fraud, and abuse.

- The administrative burden of American health care is wasteful and excessive. It diverts resources from patient care and has created mountains of paperwork for health care providers.

- Special interest groups of the medical-industrial complex have systematically taken advantage of the American people and of the complexity of the health care system to further their own financial gain.

- Insurance companies and health care providers often "blame the victims," the American people, for the system's shortcomings.

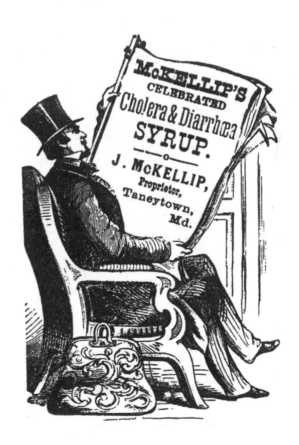

Chapter 3

The Monster II:
Perverse Incentives
Lead to Bizarre Outcomes

Mimi, a 70-year-old patient of mine who has high blood pressure, diabetes, and arthritis, came to me for a routine follow-up visit. She had seen her dermatologist, who, upon learning she had arthritis, suggested she ask her family doctor (me) for Enbrel, a new medication for arthritis. Enbrel costs over $13,000 a year, and isn't appropriate for osteoarthritis, the type she has. However, because of high demand, there is a wait list for the medication, which is used for rheumatoid arthritis.

PART OF OUR PROBLEM with overutilization comes from the demand created by physicians themselves. We have a system of perverse incentives and illogical pricing. Procedures are reimbursed generously, much more so than in other countries. And third-party reimbursement removes financial responsibility from *both* the patient and the physician.

Many specialists are prone to advise the patient to have more, as opposed to fewer, tests or procedures. Ignoring the recommendations of such bodies as the U.S. Preventive Services Task Force, they will order more frequent screening tests on the premise that they are being more thorough. Specialty organizations tend to have more generous criteria for screening that falls within the purview of their own discipline.

As opposed to the fabled "wait lists" of other countries, in America patients may have procedures or surgeries done *too* quickly. I've had patients with what I considered relatively minor complaints of knee or hip pain wind up with joint replacements the next week, even before they had a chance to do physical therapy. The otherwise healthy mother of a colleague recently was to have a knee replacement. She had a routine preoperative chest X-ray with a "spot" on it. A $5,000 PET scan ensued and the "spot" was interpreted as cancer. Lung surgery followed soon after, followed by a cascade of complications leading to her death. The pathology report showed no cancer. Then there are the hysterectomies, the tonsillectomies, a host of orthopedic procedures, and cesarean sections—many of which are not medically necessary. Maybe if we had longer "wait lists" in America, we could avoid some surgeries altogether.

There's "Gold in Them 'Thar' Patients"

AMERICAN MEDICINE HAS an amazing array of expensive "routine" diagnostic procedures, such as colonoscopy, esophagogastroduodenoscopy (looking into the stomach with a tube at $40 to $80 for each of the 26 letters in the word), MRIs for back or neck pain, prostate biopsies, sleep studies, and echocardiograms. And each specialty has its own "armamentarium" of costly procedures, the "bread and butter" of each specialist. Sometimes patients offer especially bounteous opportunities. One such gold mine comes from people who have been cooking in the sun for years to provide a crop of removable skin lesions (at $200 each) for Sunbelt dermatologists. And every pregnant woman is a potential $1,000 customer for an anesthesiologist who will place an epidural block to control her pain during labor.

Cesarean sections and epidural anesthesia during labor are two examples of a synergy between the patient and the physician that results in overutilization of expensive procedures. Patients create a demand for the procedures, even if they aren't medically necessary and may, in some circumstances, be more risky. Physicians are content to go along. After all, a cesarean section is much more convenient for the physician. It avoids being up at night as well as the stress that accompanies a long, difficult labor, and it's quicker and reimburses much more. It also removes much of the worry about malpractice should there be a problem with the baby. It would be much more appropriate to reimburse more for a difficult vaginal delivery than a cesarean section. Yet cesarean sections are reimbursed at about three times the rate of a vaginal delivery.

Epidurals are not always necessary, but patients have come to expect them. Our hospital in Nampa went for many years without anyone receiving an epidural. I think what happened was that (1) other hospitals in the area began to offer epidurals, and (2) the anesthesiologists at our hospital suddenly became willing to do them. Soon all our patients came to expect epidurals, and, even if they aren't expecting it, the nurses often convince them they need one. There's even a rush to get them done before a woman delivers! I'm not going to assert that women in labor don't need pain relief or that they categorically shouldn't have epidurals, but, given the experience of many years without the procedure, they should be used more selectively as their risk is not zero. And they can add $2,000 to the cost of a delivery.

Diagnostic tests can be very expensive. Some of the expensive ones are controversial and/or questionably necessary. For example, there is disagreement among experts as to whether liver biopsies (at $3,000) are needed for hepatitis C. And experts disagree whether it's important to follow viral counts (at $300 each) for people being treated for hepatitis C.

Unfortunately, American medicine has come to rely much more on diagnostic testing than on knowledge and cognitive thinking. It makes economic sense, since the diagnostic tests reimburse much better than cognitive efforts. I'm forced to take the cognitive approach in my everyday practice because most of my patients can't afford the tests. Ironically, by getting fewer diagnostic tests, in many cases the uninsured may be getting better care. The expensive tests often have incidental insignificant findings (now termed "incidentalomas"), which must then be tracked down and studied more, incurring increased expense and risk to the patient. Tests create their own spiral of costs and risk. I had an elderly woman with uncontrollable hypertension. A study to look at her renal arteries led to acute renal failure and a stroke, and she wound up in a nursing home. Another patient of mine, also an elderly woman, had an exam to look at her common bile duct and wound up getting pancreatitis with a full cascade of catastrophes. She spent the next 12 months in hospitals and nursing homes. In retrospect (hindsight is always easier than foresight), some patients might be better off if we had longer waiting lines for nonurgent procedures.

Relatively speaking, surgeries cost even more. And some of the newer medications, like Enbrel or Remicade for rheumatoid arthritis, can cost $13,000 to $20,000 a year.[1] New technologies have created new markets and new demands—and high prices. Emerging technologies of the future are likely to make the current "new" technologies look like bargains.

Creating the Demand: The Sky's the Limit

How REALISTIC IS IT for Americans to expect to benefit from all these new technologies? Would *not* being able to benefit from the new wonders be considered rationing? It's a dilemma. We have created a health care culture with a "sky's the limit" attitude. Corporate America and the medical profession have sold the philosophy of limitless progress to America. Employers and insurance companies have tried to put the brakes on the spending through impersonal cost-cutting approaches that have alienated the public, but no one has dealt with the "great expectations." Commercial interests, through such tactics as the direct-to-consumer ads, have only fueled the fire of rising health care costs, causing *de facto* overutilization.

I fear that we have only seen the tip of the iceberg in a geometric acceleration of these costs. As an example, what if every American with heart disease or at risk for heart disease acted upon the TV ads they saw touting Plavix (a blood thinner)? What if everyone currently on preventive doses of aspirin were switched to Plavix? For the nation as a whole, the extra cost could be 40 million at-risk people, times $111 a month for 30 Plavix pills, times 12 months a year, or over $50 billion a year just for that one drug. New research studies that come out nearly every week, like the comparison between Cozaar and atenolol for treating high blood pressure, show the advantages of newer (and much more expensive) treatments. The cost implications for the cholesterol-lowering "statin" drugs are similarly astronomical. But the "statins" appear (at least for the moment) to be a truly effective and life-saving therapy.

Meanwhile, we have strayed from the ethic of health care being a public good. Surgical procedures are patented. Inventions and new products that have a potential for improving people's health are now commercial properties. They are sold on "the market" to the highest bidders, even if many were conceived and developed with public funds. And the motivation to develop the new products comes from their profit potential rather than need. What has become of the healing ethic in health care?

The Ultimate Overutilization: "Boutique Medicine" for the Very Rich

IT'S ALMOST UNBELIEVABLE THAT, in a country where there are more than 46 million people who have no health insurance and millions who go without care because they can't afford it, we now have "boutique medicine" for the very rich.

This new phenomenon reflects the growing gap between the rich and poor. "Concierge care," as documented in an August 2001 Associated Press article, now enables millionaires to have personal primary care doctors, available on short notice at any hour. No longer does the multimillionaire need to waste time pursuing the usual paths of our dysfunctional medical system. For a price, quoted as $1,500 to $20,000 a year beyond the cost of the usual insurance, the busy executive or tycoon can have the at-the-ready presence of a primary care physician. And there's no time limit on the visit. For the physician, it can mean seeing one or two patients a day while earning more money.

The whole concept of a personal doctor for the very rich or privileged seems warped, an aberration of what a doctor is supposed to be about. When doctors' educations have been so heavily subsidized by public funding, is it ethical that they devote themselves to serving a handful of people who are willing to pay exorbitant fees for care? Speaking from the other side, don't the wealthy purchasers of these services have a right to spend their money on a product that saves their valuable time and gives them easy access to information and services they need? Yet something seems wrong when doctors themselves are treated as commodities, like a market widget, to be bought and sold.

Rich people, including kings, princes, and heads of state from around the world, have flocked to high-profile clinics in the United States to get their specialty care. And, in these days of cost-cutting managed care, their dollars have been welcomed with open arms. In some European countries with universal-coverage systems, like England and Ireland, people who want to avoid the waiting lines of the government-run systems buy private insurance and get quicker, though not necessarily better, care. Even in Canada, where there is a national commitment to equal access for services covered under the national health plan and an aversion to "jumping the queue," there is pressure from more conservative forces to privatize elements of the system and, thus, give the rich quicker access to specialist services. A few Canadians, though nowhere near the alleged "droves" in the myths,[2] do "jump the queue" and come to the United States for care.

The "concierge doctors" are perhaps one of the most outlandish developments that have occurred in our imminent transition to a multitiered health care system. They are the ultimate high-end expression of the American style of health care rationing. As the "haves" get even better access to care, the "have-nots" are finding their access to be increasingly more difficult. Even Medicare, which some conservatives seem committed to privatizing, is in imminent danger of going in this direction. The new "designer doctor" phenomenon is worrisome for several reasons. Among them:

- It reinforces the concept of health care as a commodity.

- It highlights the failure of our system to meet the genuine needs of people. As long as we do not have a working system, those who can afford it will find ways to "opt out" of the system.

- As mentioned above, it widens the gap between rich and poor, a gap that is a primary reason in itself for the overall poor health status of Americans, compared to people in other developed countries. The corollary of an expensive system for the rich is, most likely, the under-funding of care for everyone else.

Opting Out: An American Privilege?

MANY AMERICANS FEEL THAT when and if we have basic health care reform, people who can afford it should be able to opt out of the system to get "extra" services. Part of this sentiment may come from the fears of people who are satisfied with their current insurance coverage and health care. They worry that a new "national" system may dilute their benefits. This fear is one of the major stumbling blocks to health care reform. It was the primary reason that the promoters of a single-payer ballot initiative in Maryland changed their universal coverage plan to a multi-payer approach.

Perhaps there is a fair and workable way for Americans to be able to go "outside the system" in seeking their health care. Nearly all the European countries have this kind of "safety valve." And we do have a model of this kind of practice in America in the realm of education. Everyone pays taxes for schools, yet they have a choice to go to a private or parochial school at their own added expense. Hopefully, if the United States chooses to take the path of national health insurance (as I believe we should), the "plan" will be comprehensive enough and of high enough quality that people will have no need to go out-side the system for necessary services. The upcoming reform of Britain's National Health System (NHS) has provoked this very debate. In Britain, to improve their system, they foresee an increase in health care spending from about 7 percent of their GDP to 12.5 percent, with the goal of building a national con-sensus "around making the NHS the best insurance policy in the world."[3]

Closely related to the concept of "opting out" is the principle of "choice." The health care industry has given prominent atten-tion to this issue. We are told that Americans will demand "choice" and that any solution must be "pluralistic"; that is, not single payer. The rhetoric gets vague because the touted "choice" is not real choice (which would mean choice of physicians and hospitals), but choice of "plan," which paradoxically really means less choice of the more important variables: the doctors and hospitals. All plans basically restrict choice and treatment options. Even the impending new trend toward "defined-contribution" plans is headed towards less choice. As health policy expert Rima Cohen stated,[4] "Don't be fooled by calls for more choice. I think all Americans want choice of their health care providers. I don't see individuals clamoring as much for their choice of health plans, their . . . choice of benefit packages."

The "concierge doctors" represent an extreme option for the very rich to opt out of the system. Ironically, the concept of the "concierge" primary care doctor did not originate in America. The Cubans have been doing it for decades. Their system assigns a family practice doctor to about 600 people, whom that doctor follows and gets to know intimately. The difference is that the orientation is towards comprehensive care for a *community*, with a public health focus, as opposed to providing "super service" for an individual or a particular family. Maybe we can learn about community medicine from Cuba.

Competition vs. Cooperation

AFTER GIVING A TALK about health care reform at the City Club in Boise, I was asked a question about the growing competitiveness between the city's two major hospitals. In efforts to gain market share, they were duplicating services by setting up new expensive specialty units, a trend that has since continued. Now they even have competing helicopter services. I ducked the question, but I shouldn't have. It later became clear to me what was wrong. These two warring hospitals were vying for "market share." In the 1990s, financial considerations (and, for some, survival) had risen to the highest priority, even for not-for-profit hospitals, which these two hospitals are. But instead of cooperating to meet the needs of the community in the most cost-efficient way, the two hospitals took the path of competition. They chose to spend millions of dollars on costly duplication of facilities and services as well as full-page ads to compete for market share.

A front-page article in *USA Today*[5] documents how hospitals all over America are spending millions on new high-tech facilities to do expensive (and profitable) procedures, especially cardiac surgery. This competitive "arms race" reflects a lack of overall health care planning, but it is consistent with the perverse economic incentives built into our current system. These incentives give financial rewards to subspecialty operative procedures. Meanwhile, general hospitals, where many uninsured and low-income people must seek access to care, will suffer as the specialty centers draw away the paying patients. If these public hospitals, with their ERs and trauma centers, are forced to close their doors (as may soon happen in Los Angeles) because their paying patients have been diverted to for-profit subspecialty entities, the whole community will suffer.

Competition has been hawked as a way to decrease costs. Even Clinton's failed health scheme was built on faith in "the

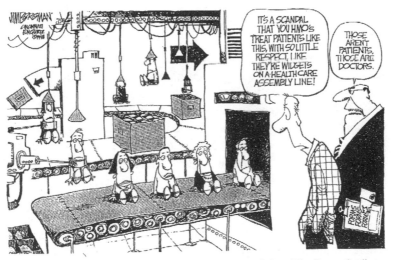

Reprinted with special permission of King Features Syndicate

market" and the unproven concept of "managed competition." I shudder with disbelief when I reflect back on the '90s and the mad scramble for "market share." Even at our local level, we had long meetings and debated for months about how to form PPOs, PHOs, HMOs, and a variety of other alphabet-soup constructs. All these schemes were aimed at preserving or expanding our "market share" of that new commodity, "covered lives." Could we have really hired consultants at $375 an hour (we did) to lead us through a maze of absurd legal constructs in which patients were reduced to mere widgets of production? Not to mention the role in the production line that physicians were being forced to assume by the managed care organizations. On the health care food chain, only patients ranked lower than physicians, while the managed care CEOs and the high-priced consultants were at the top.

Health planning has been a dirty word in America. With the demise of the old certificate of need programs, anyone desiring to open an MRI center (or other diagnostic enterprise) and sell their product on a competitive open market is free to do so. But this competitive milieu only raises overall costs because the products have to be aggressively marketed. And marketed they are, just like whole-body CAT scans or new pharmaceutical products, without regard for whether they add any value to medical care.

"The market" works in strange and illogical ways in health care. A surplus of medical subspecialists actually increases the cost of medical care, and a surfeit of new expensive technologies also increases overall costs. Instead of lowering costs through competition, the excess of doctors and technologies creates more demand. Ironically, America has many MRI machines that are so much in demand that they function almost all night long, yet there is no assurance that the MRIs ordered really improve care. And now we have PET scans at five times the price.

In health care, it makes so much more sense to make cooperation the norm. There could be standards for which diagnostic tests are appropriate and when they should be ordered. There could be improved cooperation among physicians and other health care providers instead of competition. Care could be integrated. Duplication of services could be minimized. The Kaiser model, with salaried physicians and integrated care where all the physicians communicate with one another, makes more sense. The specialist can often be less expensive than the generalist in the long run because the specialist will sometimes recognize better when an expensive test is *not* necessary. The key is cooperation. Sometimes I have a sense that we doctors are not working together as a team with the patient's good as objective number one.

On the corporate level, competition has been pretty much of a failure for health care. The "big guys" seem to have come out on top. Like the game of "Survivor," the UnitedHealthcares, the Wellpoints, and the Aetnas seem to have held their ground while smaller corporations faded. The result? An oligopoly of health plans, with less choice for consumers (aka patients in the old days).

As for the big pharmaceutical companies, they have been playing games, such as paying a competitor not to produce a drug, that make a mockery of true competition (see Chapter 1, Myth #11). Cooperation? The most notorious "cooperation" in the drug business has been the kind that can run afoul of antitrust laws. In this brand of cooperation, drug companies conspire to keep prices high, as in the vitamin scandal, for which they paid a fine of almost a billion dollars. Why couldn't cooperation involve some kind of joint efforts to produce drugs that are really needed, not look-alike drugs, such as a tenth new ACE inhibitor to treat high blood pressure?

Prevention vs. Cure

AMERICANS ARE GREAT AT coming up with quick fixes. A free clinic to help the uninsured or a bake sale to finance an operation. But we've done poorly in our long-term efforts to build a health care system that is responsive to the needs of our people. We're number one in the world for health care spending, but we rank much lower in value obtained for the amount of money spent. As mentioned earlier, our health care system came in 37th overall in the

2000 World Health Organization rankings. A major reason for our disparate performance is our failure to pay attention to prevention and public health.

Instead of doing our best to prevent chronic illnesses, like heart disease and diabetes, we develop expensive technologies to alleviate the diseases once they occur. New hearts, new lungs, new livers, new kidneys, stents in arteries, wondrous feats of medicine and surgery. But we bitterly oppose such measures as higher tobacco taxes, seat belt laws, regulations to limit pollutants, meaningful health education, and gun control. Part of the opposition comes from the American worship of individual rights, but another large part comes from corporate lobbyists who are protecting the financial interests of their industries. Public health does not have the financial clout to fight back. Prevention is lucky to get a hundredth of the resources that go to curative medicine.

A study by Yale economist William D. Nordhaus on the economic contribution of health care suggested "the social productivity of health care spending might be many times that of other spending."[6] He was looking at the increase in life expectancy at birth in the first half of the twentieth century, from 49 to 68 years. Nordhaus seemed to be suggesting that our investment in health care is not so wasteful in general economic terms. But what he fails to mention is that the great majority of the health gains in the past century came from public health measures—clean water and air, safe food, sanitation, safe working places, traffic safety, and better housing—instead of expensive medical interventions. The stent placers and joint inserters have certainly helped the quality of life for many older folks, but their overall effect on the health of the nation has been minuscule compared to what public health has accomplished.

Our health care monster, motivated by money, has given little more than lip service to prevention and public health. From the point of view of the private practitioner, who is charging hundreds or thousands of dollars each time he or she probes some orifice or removes some bit of flesh, public health is fairly irrelevant. A place to get kids' shots? Where you go if you have venereal disease or need birth control pills? Tasks with minor financial impact on the system.

Even the health maintenance organizations (HMOs), so named because they were supposed to promote prevention, have (with a few exceptions) given short shrift to prevention. They have mostly hawked prevention as an advertising tool. After all, for the HMOs, it makes little financial sense to invest in prevention when their patients, who probably will have changed insurance plans or jobs, are unlikely to be still enrolled in their plans after 3 years.

In our $2.1 trillion health care industry, little attention has been paid to such really sensible and constructive documents as *Healthy People 2010*, the U.S. Public Health Service's blueprint of health goals for America in 2010. This blueprint includes universal coverage as a goal as well as a host of accomplishments in prevention.

Our failure to resolve the problem of uninsurance in America reflects our lack of support for prevention. Because the uninsured lack access to primary care and delay their care, they develop more expensive maladies, which, if treated earlier (preventively) could have been managed for a fraction of the cost.

The Malpractice Conundrum

AMERICA IS UNIQUE AMONG the nations of the world in the prominence we have given to the issue of malpractice. Strangely enough, were we to have a more equitable system of health care that embraced universal coverage, the malpractice awards could be greatly diminished. There would be no price tag to argue over in the "medical costs" section of lawsuits. I doubt that we have more malpractice than other countries, but we do have a large amount of medical errors (that could be potential malpractice) that go unrecognized or unchallenged. Thousands of medical mistakes—wrong decisions—never come to light because people don't know any better or are not sufficiently empowered to challenge them in court. In these situations, the victims are usually obliged to pay for the mistakes of their aberrant caregivers. Call it fairness, American style.

After leveling off as an issue for several years, the issue of malpractice, at the beginning of the twenty-first century, is again becoming a major cost factor. It also affects how and where physicians practice medicine. Because of the sharp increase in the amount of malpractice awards—they now average $3.5 million compared to $1.1 million in 1994[7]—insurers have boosted their premiums. The rise in premiums has forced doctors in some states (such as West Virginia and Pennsylvania) to quit their practices. Whole geographic areas are left without adequate coverage for some specialties, such as obstetrics. Although there is great unevenness in its effects, the overall cost of malpractice to the system has been often overstated. Up to now, malpractice premiums have totaled less than 1 percent of all health care costs. "Defensive medicine" probably adds another 2 or 3 percent. But the fact that malpractice premiums are once again increasing is worrisome because care will become more expensive.

The solution probably lies in some form of no-fault malpractice insurance, except for egregious or malicious deviations. But "no-fault" would require some consensus that we are all in this society together, all at risk at some point.

The existence of the malpractice phenomenon isn't all bad. It has brought some accountability to the practice of medicine. However, its application has been uneven and often capricious, and more often than not it has been driven by opportunism and greed. As for liability and health plans, it is only just that if the plans make decisions affecting health care outcomes, they should be legally responsible and pay for their faulty judgment. Of course, the mere fact that we have a system that can argue over health "plan" liability and "patient protections" is a reflection of how far we have wandered off course on the issue of health.

Employer-Based Insurance: An Anomaly

AMERICA IS UNIQUE IN the developed world in the way in which employers control their employees' access to health insurance. Our system of employer-based health insurance came about as an economic construct of World War II, when wage controls limited the ability of employers to raise wages. As an alternative, they gave their workers health insurance. This arrangement has led to some perverse incentives. Although most employees, at least according to recent polls, seem comfortable with the system, they are generally unaware of what other arrangements could be feasible. They also are wary of change.

Health insurance has become an extension of wages and a tax-free boon for both the employer and the employee. In fact, the tax-free status of the health insurance benefit constitutes a federal bonus of about 10 percent of health care costs, estimated to be about $180 billion in 2005.

The incentives are twisted with employer-based insurance. The employer can use the insurance as a recruiting and retention tool in times of low unemployment. But if unemployment rises, there is less incentive for the employer to be generous with the insurance benefit. So, with the increasing costs of insurance, and with an economic downturn (as happened in 2001), employers can see an advantage to shifting more of the cost of insurance to employees. Employees usually accept their fate, or often they drop coverage for their dependents because they can no longer afford it. But in an extreme case, schoolteachers in Monmouth County, New Jersey, went to jail rather than accept the school district's plan to increase the employee share of the cost.

For employees, who have become accustomed to regarding health insurance through an employer as a "given," the arrangement creates even stranger incentives. People get locked into jobs, especially if a family member has a preexisting condition. They turn down opportunities that might enhance their careers or make them happier because they fear losing health insurance coverage. They endure difficult and sometimes humiliating situations.

Seeing the inequity in the system of employer-based insurance, where the interests of the employers and employees are often divergent, many organizations, such as the AMA and the American Academy of Family Physicians (AAFP), have advocated for the end of this illogical link. It is surprising that small business, which covers far fewer of its employees than big business, does not push to eliminate the connection. It puts small business at a recruiting disadvantage, while big business is able to reap the tax benefit. In a Microsoft Web site editorial, Joseph Anthony argues for small business to support universal coverage.[8]

Divorcing health insurance from being a direct work "benefit"—really wages, but not generally perceived as such—would level the playing field for business, both domestically and internationally. Foreign corporations have their employees' health insurance paid for outside the corporation, so their lower production costs mean that their American counterparts are put at an economic disadvantage. American automobile manufacturers estimate that nearly $1,400 of the cost of every vehicle that rolls off the assembly line is directly attributed to the cost of health benefits, giving Volkswagen and Toyota an automatic competitive advantage. As Robert Kuttner asks in an article that appeared in *Business Week*,[9] "When will business at last wake up, break the odd link between employment and health coverage, and support universal health insurance?"

More Perverse Incentives for Providers and Patients Alike

THE CASE OF MY patient who is experiencing "health care financing by subpoena" is almost as outlandish as going to jail over health insurance benefits:

> *Kevin is a 53-year-old man who was found to have a blockage of his lower colon when he was examined with a scope. Even barium would barely pass through the obstruction. The surgeon felt Kevin likely had colon cancer and needed surgery urgently, but Kevin hesitated. He is uninsured and has few resources. Seeking financial help, Kevin spent 2 months jumping through hoops to get our county to help pay for his surgery. They put a lien on his house. And they subpoenaed him to come to a hearing—contempt of court if he didn't show up—to decide on his case. Meanwhile, he's feeling better, has no bowel complaints, and is gaining weight. Maybe he won't need surgery. But he's had the privilege of experiencing health care financing by subpoena, just one of the ways we rob Americans of their dignity because they are poor and sick.*

As it has evolved, our nonsystem has created a plethora of perverse incentives. Health care providers and, even more tragically, people who have the misfortune to be sick have been especially affected.

Because of the lack of any overall planning, the staffing of our health care system is incredibly inefficient and unbalanced. We have an oversupply of specialists, all eager and willing to carry out the special expensive procedures they have been trained to do. And we have an undersupply of nurses and medical technicians, who, because they are in short supply in hospitals, limit the capacity of hospitals to serve patients. With increasing frequency, hospitals are being forced to close their doors to new patients or divert sick patients elsewhere because of inadequate staffing. Meanwhile, an oversupply of administrators and consultants has sprung up to manage a system that is increasingly out of control. And our system continues to have a severe geographic maldistribution of resources, largely because of perverse economic incentives. Providers in rural areas get reimbursed less than they would in urban areas for the same services, so why should someone move to a rural area, especially if he or she is leaving medical training with huge debts to pay off?

Because of their debts, physicians have much more of an incentive to become specialists to earn more money. I remember an ophthalmology professor at my medical school (Johns Hopkins) impressing us students as we watched him do cataract surgery. "That's $200 [it would be $900 to $2,000 today] for 10 minutes' work," he remarked, "and I do three of these an hour." That was when the minimum wage was a dollar an hour. Fifteen years later, I was still charging only $9 for an office visit.

The discrepancy is even worse for patients, who must suffer not only the financial consequences but also the pain and the loss of dignity. Today, if a person with a limited income does not get health insurance through an employer, the insurance will be virtually unaffordable. Should that person be sick or have a preexisting condition, the cost of the insurance, if he or she can even get insurance, will be prohibitive. Moreover, the insurance companies will force those people to face an incredibly complex set of conditions and restrictions designed to deny them the care they need. It's ironic and sad that the people who need the care most are the ones who are most penalized. They are priced out of the market.

Even if someone has an employer who provides health insurance, often the employee has to pay extra to cover a spouse or dependents. Many people find that coverage unaffordable. In the group policy at our clinic, the cost for covering a spouse and dependents is an extra $450 a month. If the take-home check is $1,000 a month, it's obvious that buying the extra coverage is impossible. And the more health care that the members of the group use, the more the insurance company will charge everyone in that group. One person's expensive illness can lead to a huge increase in premiums for everyone in a group, as happened with our clinics' health insurance in 2002. It's a vicious cycle that forces people to become "health care beggars" or go without. It's better not to get sick.

The Mental Health Scam

THE SITUATION IS EVEN worse when health problems involve mental illness. One of my patients illustrates our system's failure:

> *Ronald is a 45-year-old man who works for a major corporation in our community. His employer provides health insurance, but that insurance does not cover mental illness. Although his earnings are adequate, he incurred a huge hospital bill when he was hospitalized for a major depression. He followed up at our "safety-net" clinic because he had to pay his hospital bill himself and then couldn't afford his expensive medications.*

Mental health in the United States not only carries a stigma but is burdened with a financial penalty as well. It's amazing how much resistance we have to giving mental health "parity" status with physical health. We'll pay full-fee for coronary artery bypasses or heart transplants, but insurers balk at covering depression or bipolar disorders. Is it the old "bootstraps" mentality or "personal responsibility" dogma that causes this disconnect? Or the feeling that we're personally responsible for our own mental health, whereas our failure to eat and exercise properly doesn't count against us? Remarkably, only a few years ago, the first "ER" for Idahoans with a mental health crisis was the jail.

I know we've been duped when some of my colleagues ask, "What are you going to do with mental health counselors who want to have their patients come back every day for treatment?" My reply is, of course: the same thing we should do with providers who want to do expensive sleep studies or treat heartburn with Nexium. We need to have scientifically based guidelines. But the line of questioning from my colleagues indicates that the "merchants of myth" have done their job well. Taking advantage of a public bias against mental illness, insurers have persisted in resisting parity for mental illness. They have convinced business to oppose parity by using the timeworn mantra that parity "would increase the costs of health insurance and lead to more uninsured." All the evidence, however, points to a minimal increase in costs, not to mention the inherent inequity in ascribing a less scientific basis to major mental illness than to coronary artery disease. And, if we look at the cost to society as a whole, I would suspect that the adequate treatment of mental illness and substance abuse problems in America would save our society billions of dollars. Likely there would be fewer school massacres, teen suicides, people "going postal," and drug- and alcohol-related disasters. Another advantage (often overlooked) is the millions of dollars a year that could be saved if individuals incarcerated in our jails and penitentiaries for anger-related crimes and drug addiction were instead treated in outpatient clinics with appropriate psychiatric and medical management, not to mention returning those individuals to society as productive citizens. We might even see fewer anthrax-laced letters. Veteran TV commentator Mike Wallace (who has had a major problem with depression) eloquently expresses the dilemma in an op-ed piece, entitled "Mind and Body," that appeared in *The New York Times*.[10]

The real culprit here is money. The insurance companies are taking advantage of the situation to minimize their "medical losses." Just as they delay payment to physicians for as long as possible to retain capital for their own use, they are trying to delay the inclusion of mental health benefits for as long as possible. Meanwhile, even people who have insurance that covers mental illness or treatment for substance abuse find their coverage limits them to incredibly inadequate amounts of care, such as 2 or 3 weeks a year of inpatient therapy. I'd like to see an insurance company argue *for* mental health parity. Then I'd know they were putting the interests of Americans first.

The Patient Comes Last

ATTENTION TO THE NEEDS of the patient should come first, not last. Symbolically, however, America has come to place the interests of patients at the bottom of the list, whereas the "bottom line" has assumed a place at the top. Some health care gurus, like Paul Ellwood, whose name has been invoked as one of the promoters of the "managed-care revolution," are now advocating that America reverse course. Ellwood, in a speech calling for "HEROIC" changes, says, "The emphasis should be on the health component rather than financial incentives."[11] He doesn't go quite far enough. In fact, he partially misses the point by not placing the patient, or at least the "health of the patient," instead of the "health system" at the top of the list. His "R" portion of "HEROIC" seems to reinforce our health system's proclivity towards "blaming the victim"; that is, the patient. He wants patients to "assume greater responsibility for their own health and for the cost of the health care that they require."[12]

Physicians have often been critical of patients "who abuse the system," as related in Chapter 2 (the "overutilizers"). There is certainly a level at which "personal responsibility" should play a role. But the cards are so stacked against the patients in our system (an article published in *Health Affairs* in 2005 revealed that more than 50 percent of bankruptcies are medically related; the majority of them were middle-class people, 75 percent of whom actually had health insurance when they got sick) that the mantra of "personal responsibility" is like asking a school of naive minnows to swim in a sea full of sharks. Instead of complaining about the misuse of ERs, our system should be adapting more to meet the needs of people seeking care.

As for the drinkers, smokers, and overeaters, the solution goes beyond the health care system. It involves society as a whole. It behooves health care professionals to leave our safe little havens in the health system to venture out into the political and societal arena. That's where we should be advocating for the changes that can deal more globally with the issue of self-abusive habits. We need to remember that all of us exhibit some risky behaviors at one time or another. Should the downhill skier who hits a tree be required to pay her or his own medical bills?

Discrimination against people who are sick or who have chronic diseases is a much larger, and serious, issue. It's the cardinal rule of how the insurance game is played and of how the system games the sick: avoid risk. From the insurance companies' viewpoint, avoiding risk (people who are sick and, therefore, potentially more expensive) is the key to staying profitable. In our nation approximately 20 percent of the people consume 80 percent of the health care dollars. In dollar terms, the average annual health care expenses per person in this top 20 percent exceeds $28,000 compared to the average overall cost of about $7,000.[13] Any accountant can figure out that avoiding this high-risk group and insuring only people who are well is the goal. For people with a to-be-avoided preexisting condition, insurers either refuse to cover them or charge a fortune for coverage. I have a patient (a single woman in her fifties with generalized muscle weakness) who lost her job and is running out of COBRA coverage.[14] She got a quote of $1,000 a month from a major insurer. Many people are afraid to use their health insurance because they fear their coverage will be canceled. Personal responsibility for patients? How about corporate responsibility, some obligation to the communities they serve, for the insurance companies?

In the debates about health care, little attention has been paid to the needs of the patient. Maybe this anomaly has come about because of the false perception that it isn't the patient who pays for the insurance. The assumption is that it's the employer who is purchasing the coverage and is therefore entitled to call the shots. The employee, whose health insurance is really part of his or her wage compensation, is getting short shrift. There are national arguments over the business practices of health plans, controlling costs for employers, or cutting back on the Medicaid spending of state governments. Relatively little public discussion goes into the issue of holding down costs for employees or patients. In fact, as alluded to above, the trend clearly seems to be to find innovative new ways to shift more costs to employees/patients. In the shadow of a market where the costs of health care and premiums are rising rapidly (outpacing the growth of our economy on average by a factor of 3), many employees/patients will likely be priced out of the market.

The Market vs. the Patient

DESPITE THE MORE GENERAL acceptance recently that "the market" does not fit health care in the same way in which it applies to other economic enterprises, the market rhetoric—now morphed to "empowering the patient" and "choice"—continues. Unfortunately, for many people of limited means, the kind of increased "choice" promoted in the new "defined-contribution" schemes may be the choice to forgo needed health care.

The failure of the market in health care, with the demise of managed care as we knew it, came about largely because of its failure to recognize that people were not just widgets. When people (and physicians) finally caught on to how they were being abused by managed care, they rebelled. And "the market" in health care, at least as we knew it, collapsed. Or, perhaps more alarmingly, it may be in a state of metamorphosis. We seem to be on a path, with new euphemisms, that still leaves the patient at the bottom of the priority list.

The dilemma of organizing "patient power" to come up with a patient-friendly solution, versus an employer or corporate-friendly solution, is daunting. Conservative belief/rhetoric promotes corporate growth with the assumption that a prosperous corporate America will mean "more jobs," with improved worker status (the old "trickle-down" theory). Whenever I see the words "more jobs," I immediately translate the phrase into "more profits," just as I translate that other conservative mantra, "personal responsibility," into "everyone for himself." The patients/employees are behind the "rhetorical eight ball" in America. Any plea for equity, justice, or fairness in health care is countered by the cry of "socialized medicine."

How can we make sure that we meet the needs of the employee/patient? The AMA proposal for health care reform, which uses the rhetoric of "empowering patients," sounds positive. It does take an important step forward by doing away with the employer-based purchase of insurance. However, in the AMA model, the insurance industry, the pharmaceutical companies, the hospitals, and the doctors remain in control. The "monster" survives. Merely allowing more choice of plan or provider without changing the system still leaves people at the mercy of the medical-industrial complex.

Unless we deal with all aspects of our "monster," we will not succeed in meeting the needs of our people. Until we deal with the myths, put the pursuit of profit where it belongs (in "widget" industries, not health care), and place the interest of the patient first instead of last, we will not be able to fix our system and return dignity to health care. Meanwhile, we will experience an expansion of health care rationing, American style: delayed care.

Summary of Key Points

- Our employer-based health insurance system is outmoded, illogical, and needs to be replaced.

- Perverse incentives make our health care system a poor value for the amount we spend.

- Cooperation, not competition, will make health care affordable for all.

- Our nation has ignored prevention, thus creating a "time bomb" for the future.

- We need to put the patient first—not last—in the setting of priorities.

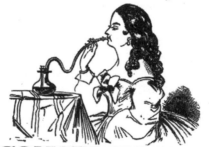

Inhaling Medicated Air into the Lungs to Cure

CONSUMPTION,
AND ALL DISEASES OF THE

THROAT AND LUNGS,

FOR INFORMATION ENQUIRE AT THE

PULMONARY INSTITUTE,
323 West Fourth Street,
CINCINNATI, OHIO.

Persons at a distance desiring treatment can have it sent by mail or express to all parts of the United States or Canada. For terms and information respecting treatment, send or write for a circular. Address

DR. N. B. WOLFE,
P. O. Box 399.

Chapter 4

Delayed Care:
Rationing American Style

Ralph is a 37-year-old man who has uncontrolled diabetes and no health insurance. He is unable to work more than a few days at a time because of chronic back problems. Although his mother, who is also a diabetic, has offered to pay for his diabetes medications and his clinic visits, he is too proud to accept the help. He only shows up at our clinic when he has an acute illness, an injury, or is in need of hospitalization.

"One reason people dismiss the problem of the uninsured is that they don't believe people are turned away. They're right. What happens is people delay getting care. And when they get it, they are more expensive to treat."[1]
—Drew Altman, President of the
Kaiser Family Foundation

LUKE, A 60-YEAR-OLD out-of-work computer programmer with diabetes, pulled a handful of change out of his pocket. "That's all I've got to last me the rest of the month, doc," he told me. "I ran out of glucose strips last week, and I can't afford to buy any more until I get my [disability] check next month." Luke was in the habit of delaying his care because he didn't always have the money and was too proud to ask for charity care, even at our health center, which has a "nominal" fee for visits. Two years ago he went a little too long without care for his diabetes and wound up having two toes amputated.

93

Gwen, a woman in her forties who works part-time at a "big-box" store, had a severe intestinal illness with a high fever. She came in after 5 days, and I asked why she had waited so long to seek care. "Because I still owed you $6," she replied. She came in after she got her meager paycheck for $37 that allowed her to pay off the first bill.

Defenders of our current health care system tout the myth that everyone in America, including the uninsured, has access to care through the emergency rooms (see Chapter 1, Myth #1), so there's no health care crisis (Myth #2). The uninsured are not hurting. Yet nearly every epidemiological study done on health care in America has shown that the uninsured have much higher morbidity and mortality than the insured.[2] The discrepancy, moreover, is not just related to social class or economic status. Put bluntly, the uninsured, even middle-class Americans, delay or avoid care because they literally cannot afford it. And, when they finally come in for care, they're sicker and more expensive to treat.

We have rationing of health care in America. Those Americans who worry about the rationing of care, if America should move towards a health care system like Canada's or Great Britain's, can relax. We already have it, American style. It's a simple formula. If you can afford the care, you can get it; if not, you can't. The American formula for rationing is particularly unfriendly to the uninsured. They even pay more for services than the insured, as described above (see Chapter 1, Myth #9). They are billed full fee for every service they consume. People with insurance, however, usually are billed at a discounted rate that was negotiated by their managed-care plans. However, even the insured are being increasingly priced out of the market, despite their insurance, because of the ever-growing size of deductibles and co-pays. And it looks like there will be more self-imposed rationing in the near future.

Higher out-of-pocket costs are all but a certainty as businesses move toward "defined contributions" or so-called "consumer-driven" health care. Even Medicaid patients may soon have to pay previously outlawed co-pays. States trying to control run-away Medicaid expenditures may soon be able to obtain waivers from the federal government to impose co-pays on beneficiaries—co-pays that in effect will ration care. The shortsightedness is frightful. The system is looking at short-term fiscal impact instead of considering the long-term effects. The lack of insurance or the imposition of higher co-pays only leads to delayed care. It's true that medical care is not really necessary for some self-limited conditions, such as colds, minor muscular strains, or "intestinal flu." But the delayed care for chronic conditions (like diabetes, high blood pressure, asthma, or depression) costs the individual and society much more in the long run. The example of my patient Ralph, the 37-year-old diabetic, is illustrative. A recent study examining the factors related to poor outcomes in diabetics found that "lack of insurance was the most consistent correlate of inadequate care."[3] We all pay for the costs of catastrophes like kidney failure, heart attacks or strokes, either through cost-shifting (as with the uninsured) or premium increases (for the insured). Delayed care is costly for everyone.

The Mantra of "Personal Responsibility"

SO WHY DOES OUR SOCIETY tolerate financial barriers that lead to delayed care when it would be so much more cost-effective to design a system that encourages timely care, not to mention the adverse human effects? We have created an ethos, and many people actually believe it, that we don't value something we don't pay for. The corollary to this philosophy would be that the more we pay for something, the more we think it's worth. For the uninsured, they're simply priced out of the market and they won't seek care unless they're in dire straits.

The insured are now being sold the myth that somehow it's better that they have more responsibility to share in the cost of their care. The mantra of "personal responsibility" is being invoked to cover the failures of the system. It's as if paying more for your health care somehow builds character. Meanwhile, the costs to patients have increased so much that even the insured often must delay care for lack of affordability. What is their insurance for? Don't they realize that with insurance they are already paying in advance for their health care? It's not free. Even if their

employers are picking up the entire cost of the insurance, and
that's getting to be an almost nonexistent situation these days,
those premiums are really part of their salaries. For the federal
programs, we have all paid up front for the services received
through taxes, taxes that we paid in advance. That's the meaning
of insurance. But the insurers want us to pay extra so that we will
hesitate to use the services, even when they're needed or prudent
to use.

Low-income people must make economic choices, and paying for health care is one of those choices. Although some state
legislators envisage the uninsured as choosing between buying a
second snowmobile or health insurance, that example is ludi-
crous. The uninsured people I see are choosing between paying
the rent, buying food, or paying for their lab tests and medicines.
They often don't come in because they haven't got enough
money to buy gasoline to get to the clinic. A recent op-ed column
in *The New York Times* by Bob Herbert on hunger[4] alluded to "the
elderly look[ing] wistfully at food on television—food they can't
have because they spend their money on their medicine."

Some Terrible Consequences of Delayed Care

HERE ARE A FEW MORE EXAMPLES of delayed care—and its
consequences—in people we have seen at our community health
center:

1. A 24-year-old uninsured single mother of two who is very
   ill with fevers and weakness, delays coming in for a few
   days because she is afraid of the bill. She dies the next day
   with a bacterial infection of her heart valves.

2. A 29-year-old uninsured married mother of two who skips
   prenatal care because she can't afford even our discounted
   fees. She comes to the hospital 2 weeks overdue with a dead
   12-pound baby; she herself dies of a complication of pregnancy (amniotic fluid embolus) as she's about to get a
   cesarean section.

3. A 63-year-old man with heart disease and hypertension, who delays coming in for 3 months because he owes us $12. He runs out of medicine, goes into severe congestive heart failure, and needs to be hospitalized.

4. The 16-year-old uninsured son of a clinic employee (we don't pay for dependents' insurance) who injures his ankle while he's away at camp. Care is delayed, the ankle is broken, and more costly treatment is necessary.

5. A 54-year-old uninsured man with a severe lung problem who is to follow up with a specialist but gives up on the system because he is asked to pay a large sum up front before he is seen. He doesn't return until 3 months later after having lost 40 pounds. He then requires hospitalization and rehabilitative therapy for 6 months for what turned out to be pulmonary tuberculosis.

6. A man in his early sixties with diabetes who had been followed at another clinic until he lost his health insurance after an injury on his job. Although his ophthalmologist continued to see him and do five eye surgeries, he stopped getting medical care for his diabetes 2 years ago and ran out of his diabetes medications a year and a half ago. He came in with his diabetes way out of control (his blood sugars in the 300s) and kidney failure. He had worked his entire life until his accident 2 years ago.

I see delayed care and its short- and long-term negative (and costly) effects on a daily basis. It's sad from the viewpoint of both economic waste and human suffering. The results are not always as catastrophic as in the examples above. Often the conditions get better by themselves, without a medical intervention. Sometimes the delays are of a preventive nature, such as the 35-year-old mother who just had her fourth baby and is unable to afford a tubal ligation because she doesn't have the up-front payment. We expect to see her back soon with her fifth pregnancy.

But there are so many situations, especially with chronic diseases and neglected injuries, where the end result of delayed care is disastrous and/or very costly. There are also the people whom we don't even see, who suffer silently because they won't come in. Although people have an array of reasons for not seeking care, the financial barrier ranks highest in their decision to delay or omit care. These Americans can be compared to many poor people in third-world countries, who can't even imagine being able to get the care they need. As a 45-year-old single mother told me when she brought in her daughter, "I have to set my priorities. I'll pay for my children's care, but I can't afford to get the care I need. [She needed to see an orthopedist for surgery.] I've learned to live with the pain." And so have millions of other Americans who are forced to delay care because of our failing nonsystem of health care financing. We already have rationing of health care in America—and it's getting worse. The next chapter will describe some of the makeshift strategies used by America's "safety-net" providers to try to cope with a system that forces patients to delay care.

A postscript:

Ralph, the 37-year-old uninsured diabetic referred to at the beginning of this chapter, came back to our clinic in November 2001. He had suddenly gone blind from diabetes—retinal bleeding. With the catastrophe, he immediately got attention from an ophthalmologist who did laser surgery on his eyes (cost of about $5,000). Unfortunately, the surgery helped very little, if at all. A blood test drawn when he came in showed he was in severe kidney failure from his diabetes. His creatinine was 16.9, his creatinine clearance 1 milliliter per minute (both extremely abnormal). We had no trouble getting him hospitalized and evaluated by a kidney specialist. He is now getting dialysis and waiting for a kidney transplant. Since he needs dialysis, he will soon qualify for Medicare. Finally he gets his health insurance.

Summary of Key Points

• Rationing of health care already exists in America in the form of delayed care.

• Delayed care leads to more illness, disability, and death as well as much higher costs in the long run.

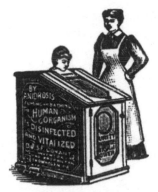

Chapter 5

Jumping Hoops for the Uninsured: Caring for Patients at a Community Health Center

Imelda is a 36-year-old mother of two who is in the third trimester of her pregnancy when she starts to have heavy vaginal bleeding. Because she is afraid of the bill, she waits 2 hours in the hospital parking lot while she bleeds profusely with a placenta previa (a placenta that covers the internal opening of the cervix). She has a cesarean section and develops a blood clot in her leg after the surgery. She is sent home with a prescription for coumadin, a blood thinner used to prevent the blood clot from going to her lung (which can be fatal). She doesn't get the prescription filled because she can't afford it.

THE SEPTEMBER 2000 "CONSUMER REPORTS" lead article entitled "Second-Class Care"[1] outlines what happens to America's uninsured when they develop serious illnesses. It especially spotlighted our "safety-net" clinics, the Community and Migrant Health Centers, and the difficulties we have getting diagnostic tests and specialty care for the patients we see. Perhaps I should be offended at being accused of giving "second-class care," but I think the article was referring not so much to the quality of care delivered at our clinics, but to the type of care that the uninsured in America receive in general. Robert L. Ferrer gives an even more graphic and disturbing account of the plight of the uninsured at his county hospital walk-in clinic in Texas. He relates his story in an opinion piece, "Within the System of No-System," that appeared in the *Journal of the American Medical Association.*[2] Our "safety-net" clinics are like putting a finger, or perhaps several fingers, in a dike (the American health care system) that has thousands of

100

leaks. Conversely, our "safety nets" could be described as a hodgepodge of leaky buckets.

Caring for the uninsured is a mix of frustration and reward with good doses of hand-holding, puzzle-solving, critical scientific thinking, and penny-pinching. It requires being a real clinician, which means also being a friend and an advocate for each patient, not just a technician. A quick history and examination, followed by a brief explanation and a prescription handed to the patient, is not sufficient.

For the past 30 years, I have been working at a community health center (CHC) whose primary purpose is to meet the needs of the uninsured. We've helped thousands of people whose contact with the health care system would otherwise be limited to showing up at ERs with a serious injury or illness.

Why They Don't Come In

PERHAPS THE GREATEST FRUSTRATION for a clinician caring for the uninsured is the lack of appropriate follow-up. Seeing an uncontrolled diabetic who comes in once every 2 years, and who ran out of medicines a year ago, is not satisfying health care. Why don't they come in? The answer would seem to be obvious, and it mostly is obvious: the lack of money. We do ask for a nominal fee (currently $10, though some other community health centers charge $20), and many patients cannot afford it. Some cannot afford even the $5 minimum fee we ask for a prescription. The fact that the prescription would cost $150 if they were to buy it at an outside pharmacy is irrelevant. I also have patients who don't want to return because they know they will need lab tests, and those will cost money. Many of the newer medications require periodic blood tests to monitor possible liver damage. Often, patients will bargain with me not to do lab tests. "Doc, I can't afford them."

But for some the failure to return for follow-up care goes beyond the lack of money. The reasons can be complex, but are rooted in the culture of poverty, something difficult for us clinicians to understand. In my state of Idaho, there are legislators who equate poverty with irresponsibility: "Those poor people should be out there finding good jobs, saving their money, and buying health insurance—not wasting their money on tobacco and VCRs." Yet, how many of us clinicians, or legislators, for that matter, have had to live with dunning by collection agencies, having our phones disconnected for nonpayment, or being grilled by a medical receptionist about our lack of insurance coverage? Or, worse, worrying about how we were going to be able to buy food for our children or pay our rent so we won't be evicted?

The stories about low-income seniors choosing between medications and food are true. That's why some of my patients stretch out their diabetes and blood pressure medications, taking them only two or three times a week instead of daily. And they come in 3 months late for their follow-up visits with blood sugars over 300 and blood pressures of 160/110. Wanting to avoid the cost and/or inconvenience of a return appointment, they often call in hoping to get their prescriptions renewed when sometimes they haven't been seen for over a year. It's frustrating for us clinicians.

When I ask my patients why they didn't return when I asked them to come back (my note on the chart clearly reads that they were to come back in 3 months), their first response is usually that they were "feeling well." Probing a little more deeply, I find the financial consideration "I didn't have the money" is nearly always a major consideration. But often it's more. It's sometimes a trade-off between work and health care. Either they can't get off work to come in, or being off work means lost wages or even fear of losing a job. Sometimes they don't come in because they're afraid we'll find something bad, and that might require more tests or X-rays that are likely to be even more costly. Then there's the wait at the clinic, and the fear that they will not be treated well or asked for money they do not have.

Pride is important. Many patients have told me—some even break down in tears in front of me—that they are ashamed to come in because they have no money to pay. It's hard for them to face emotional collapse when someone asks them for payment. They'd rather do without the health care.

I saw a woman in her thirties who was getting her Depo-Provera shots (for birth control) at the local health department because they cost less there. She had missed her shot by 3 weeks and was running a risk of getting pregnant again. I asked her why she hadn't gone back in time for her shot. She explained that the health department accepted whatever she could afford as payment. There was no set fee. But her husband was out of work and they had huge medical bills, so she didn't have any money at all. She felt ashamed to get the shot if she couldn't contribute at least $10 to the cost of her care.

For many of the reasons elaborated above, people put up with whatever condition they have. They learn to live with the pain. And then there is the whole issue of transportation, which is much more difficult in a rural area. No money for gasoline, the car broke down, my stepson ran the car into a tree, the husband drives and uses the car to get to work. So they're not there for the appointment. They often either have no phone or have had their phone disconnected, so they don't reschedule and we can't reach them easily to remind them to come in.

The Medical Visit, Prescriptions, and Tests: Games We Play

TRADITIONALLY, THE MOST FRUSTRATING obstacle for clinicians, and the most practical barrier for patients, has been obtaining needed medications. A medical visit does little good if, at the end of the visit, the patient gets a prescription he or she cannot fill. At our health center, we've managed to solve this problem the great majority of the time. Since we opened 30 years ago, we have included pharmacy services, and a pharmacist, as an integral part of our program. We have a formulary and can obtain many drugs at very reasonable prices. We even have an almost full-time person who coordinates all the paperwork to get expensive drugs for patients through indigent drug programs. More than 1,000 of our patients get their drugs through these pharmaceutical company arrangements. Other "safety-net" clinics are not so fortunate. They often work with samples or vouchers that patients take to an outside pharmacy to get drugs. To their credit, though it's not clear that their efforts are totally voluntary, the pharmaceutical companies have been supplying many of their expensive drugs to low-income people who cannot afford them. Pfizer's "Sharing the Care" program is one such arrangement that applies specifically to CHCs, including our own.

America's community health centers serve only about 10 percent of America's uninsured, although they have recently begun to receive increased funding so that they can reach twice as many people in 5 years. For the other 90 percent of the uninsured, who currently do not know about or have access to a CHC, the situation can be much more difficult. Even for a middle-income person who is self-employed or working for a small business, and who has a preexisting condition that makes buying health insurance prohibitively expensive, it's difficult to afford medications. Filling prescriptions for three common drugs like Prilosec, Lipitor, and Norvasc would cost about $400 a month. The affordability of drugs is becoming an ever-increasing problem not just for the uninsured, but for the insured as well. Seniors (with Medicare) who come to our "safety-net" clinics face the same problems if we can't get them the drugs at a reduced price. Our cut-rate prices (and the indigent drug programs) only apply to low-income people. If someone earns over 100 or 200 percent of poverty (depending on the program), they're out of luck—no discount. Even for a person at 200 percent of poverty,[3] $400 a month out of pocket for drugs is a lot of money, and sometimes the drugs cost much more.

For physicians, one of the most frustrating aspects of practicing medicine is the so-called "noncompliant" patient, the patient who didn't follow instructions or take the prescribed medicine. With soaring deductibles and co-pays for visits and (especially) drugs, physicians outside the "safety net" will soon get a taste of what it feels like to practice medicine where patient compliance is a fickle hope, where the physician must ask routinely, "Can you afford this prescription?" Physicians will feel stronger about the need to overhaul how we finance health care when they see more of their patients fail to improve because they couldn't afford the prescribed tests or medications. Of course, since many patients are too proud to say that they didn't get the medications because they couldn't afford them, the physician may never know. I have a woman in her late fifties with breast cancer who went for over a year without her tamoxifen (for preventing a recurrence) while her cancer doctor (and I, as well) thought she was taking it.

Most "safety-net" clinics have arranged access to lab tests at a fairly reasonable cost. At our center, access to such tests is no problem, unless they're expensive tests, like a quantitative viral count for hepatitis C. But many patients are still wary of lab tests. They have a hard time affording even the minimal lab fees we tack on their bill. It's even more difficult for them to pay the bills that the outside labs send them directly. At our center, our patients have "in-house" access (at reduced fees) to basic X-rays and a few common procedures, such as colposcopy (an exam of the cervix) and obstetrical ultrasound. Other clinics are not always so lucky, and their uninsured patients must often fend for themselves in paying for these tests. As clinicians, we can order a test (like a chest X-ray to be done at the hospital), but then the patient must come up with the cash to pay for it as well as the separate bill they'll get from the radiologists for reading the X-rays.

A Patchwork of Arrangements to Get Care

WHEN IT COMES TO diagnostic procedures, the situation gets much more difficult for both the clinician and the patient. Over the years, like other clinics, we've come up with a variety of piece-meal solutions that sometimes are wonderful for our patients but are often short-lived. An example is free eye exams for diabetics, but they need to be completed before the end of the month when that specific grant expires. These solutions have largely depended on a patchwork of grants, all of which require time and resources to apply for and administer. The paperwork is often lengthy and frustrating, but the patients do benefit.

The availability of mammograms is a prime example of the chaos that could be simplified if we had universal coverage in America instead of our current hodgepodge of financing. Up until about 3 years ago, only about 40 percent of our patients who needed screening mammograms actually got them. This number was undoubtedly less for the uninsured. "I don't need it, I feel well," they would say, or "I've heard they hurt," or they seemed too modest to have one. But then we got a grant from the Komen Foundation to cover mammograms for women between ages 40 and 49. And we got funding from the Women's Health Check program—with scads of intricate and frustrating administrative requirements—to cover mammograms for uninsured women between ages 50 and 64. Suddenly the same women who were saying "no" to mammograms were now saying "yes." Shame and fear of the loss of dignity create a host of excuses, which disappear when financial barriers are removed.

When our local hospital decided that it needed to do more charity care, it offered to do free or discounted diagnostic tests (the hospital part of the billing only) for our center's low-income patients. Suddenly our patients could afford to get abdominal and pelvic ultrasounds, spine X-rays, even CAT scans. MRIs, however, were not included since they belonged to a different billing entity. With the free diagnostic tests, we have to warn our patients that they will get a separate full-price bill from the radiologists, but at least we're able to get tests that patients had refused to get in the past. Unfortunately, our situation is exceptional, and most community health centers (and their patients) must continue to contend with the same barriers to diagnostic testing that we had prior to this special arrangement.

Of course, our patients are still in a quandary if they need some other expensive testing, such as colonoscopy (an examination of the colon) or angiograms (injecting dye into the arteries of the heart to see if there's a blockage). Talk about "rationing" in other countries. We have rationing U.S. style, a step below the "wait-lists" of countries like Canada and Great Britain. For non-emergency chronic conditions, many patients simply don't get the tests done until they qualify for Medicare (by waiting until they're 65) or Medicaid (which can be very difficult for an adult to do). Only if the condition is acute or life-threatening will it get taken care of right away. Then the financial damage gets sorted out later, often through collection agencies.

Sometimes the condition isn't immediately life-threatening, but it seems sufficiently apparent that a test or a procedure is really important to be done in a timely manner. Then the caregiver and the patient, with the help of people like social workers, explore the options to secure financing. County indigent funding, service club grants (for example, with eye surgery), applying for Medicaid, and asking—begging?—for charity care from the specialist are a few of the possibilities. So we play games, games that require a lot of time from a lot of people.

A case example:

> *Mary is a 64-year-old woman who was found to have "severe dysplasia" (almost cancer) on her Pap test. She is referred to a gynecologist who recommends a hysterectomy. Because she is uninsured, she spends 3 months "jumping through hoops" to secure a promise from the county to pay for her surgery. She must pay back the county $30 a month "for the rest of her life," she calculates. Had she waited 8 months longer, she would have qualified for Medicare, but by then she may have developed cervical cancer.*

"Begging, borrowing, and stealing" is what we must often do to get the needed care for our patients. Personal contact (such as between the referring clinician and the specialist) becomes the key link in the process. The referring clinicians develop relationships with individual specialists who are willing to help out and/or who have a social conscience. Unfortunately, there is often some negative fallout for these "good-guy" specialists (if they can be found, and, at least for us, they usually can, though it has become more difficult). They are often admonished by their business managers for not bringing in enough revenue, in contrast to their partners who are less willing to donate their services to indigent patients. And the "good guys" soon have their practices overwhelmed by nonpaying patients, who are often difficult and time-consuming. Several of the "good guys" in our community have recently started to decline seeing our uninsured or Medicaid patients.

Our hospital in Nampa is hurt financially by its willingness to serve our low-income patients. Since our physicians use and refer mostly to our local hospital (the other three hospitals in the area are too far away for our docs to provide efficient coverage), our hospital gets a disproportionate share of the charity care. The hospital radiologists (who bill separately from the hospital) have been hurt by having to serve our patients, who cannot afford to pay. As a result, the radiologists get paid less (the same could apply to other specialists), and the hospital has been losing radiologists to the other hospitals, where they get paid more. A vicious cycle. Or justice in health care, American style.

Why Do Our Patients Think We Don't Have Universal Coverage?

IN AN ATTEMPT TO figure out why the uninsured are not rising up in protest to demand universal coverage, I carried out a mini-survey at my clinic. I did a very seat-of-the-pants variety of qualitative research using about 100 of the patients I saw in mid-2001. Selection was based on whether there was time enough to ask the survey question. I asked only one question, though I found I had to couch it in a certain way or it could be misinterpreted. Without attempting to influence their response, I posed the following situation: "All the other developed nations of the world, like the European countries, have made sure that everyone in their countries is covered by some kind of health insurance. The United States has not. Why do you think we haven't done it? Why are we different?"

Taking into account multiple responses, 33 percent of the people included "We can't afford it" and 20 percent said they didn't know why. The next highest reasons given, in order of frequency, were: "Doctors don't want it" (14 percent), "Government doesn't care" (12 percent), and "Politics" (10 percent). There were some who "didn't trust the government" (9 percent) and faulted "greed" (also 9 percent). The specific targets of the "greed" respondents were the doctors, the insurance companies, the drug companies, and politicians. Strangely enough, an equal number (6 percent each) cited: (1) the "fear of socialized medicine" and (2) the opinion that "we should have socialized medicine." A few of the more colorful responses:

- From a 70-year-old diabetic woman: "If they're doing it in other countries, we should do it here. We're the richest country."

- From a 48-year-old uninsured woman: "Too many doctors need to have a great big Mercedes."

- From a 67-year-old woman: "Too many hypocrites in the Senate that don't care. They think of themselves and not the poor guy who can't afford it."

- From a Hispanic woman in her fifties, formerly uninsured: "We let it go by. Before we were dumb. If you were sick, [you were told] 'stay home and rest and the next day get up and go to work.' "

- From a woman in her sixties: "The insurance companies have a good deal going. They do well from those who can pay, and not by those who can't."

- From a 52-year-old woman: "Insurance companies [are] the ruination of this country."

- From an 85-year-old man: "Health insurance should be like a standing army, protecting us physically."

- From a 62-year-old Hispanic woman who always brings me tamales: "We need to unite, get together and demand [universal coverage]."

Obviously, there is a lot of resentment, a strong feeling that the uninsured have been neglected and even taken advantage of. But many people, especially those who are the poorest, have accepted the fact that they're not insured. They've written it off as something unaffordable, and they aspire toward finding a job that includes insurance coverage. They haven't given the issue much thought. I have the feeling, however, that if asked, my patients could come up with some good ideas on how to remedy our system's shortcomings. They should be given the opportunity to have their voices heard.

The Positive Side of Working With the Uninsured

THERE ARE SOME REWARDING ASPECTS of serving the uninsured. We have an incentive to avoid unnecessary tests and procedures. We must be cost-efficient in what we do because our resources—not to mention the resources of the patients—are limited. If we spend our limited budgets unwisely, we will be able to serve fewer people in need. That same motivation drives us to practice a more scientific brand of medicine. We also tend to stress prevention more, out of economic necessity as well as a perspective that (we hope) sees the larger picture. Our chronic disease "collaboratives," in which we have an organized approach to chronic disease, are examples of our efforts to join prevention with scientific outcome-based medicine.

We essentially work within a budget, and although cost is not our primary motivator (the well-being of the patient is), cost affects what we can do. Our diabetic patients don't have insulin pumps. They have a hard time affording the glucose testing strips that cost one or two dollars a day. But we do arrange free machines to test blood sugars, discounted medications, diabetic teaching, and (sometimes) scholarships for a diabetic training course. The "art" of medicine is important for us.

Uninsured patients don't expect to get every possible new test or procedure. They don't come in asking for an MRI for their back pain. They're willing to go with conservative therapeutic approaches first, so we see less iatrogenic (doctor-caused) disease. Also, we have many very grateful patients who appreciate the care we give them. Because we provide easier access to care, we're able to give better continuity of care, thus meeting more of the needs of our uninsured (or now, increasingly, underinsured) patients. Since we need to be more involved in their personal lives to be able to get them the care they need, many patients develop a more personal bond to the clinic and to our clinicians.

Outreach workers and case managers allow us to work "off-site" with the patients as well as add a more personal touch. Unfortunately, the relatively high turnover of our clinicians (at least in the past) has diminished some of the continuity. And the degree of chaos in our patients' (and their families') lives directly affects how our clinics function (sometimes also with a high degree of chaos). We are forever seeking creative solutions to meet the needs of our patients and our communities.

Community health centers have gone a long way to serving the "left-out" populations of the uninsured and (now) underinsured. But we're like a handful of fingers in a dike that is leaking badly through thousands of holes. In a recent study done by the Urban Institute, the authors found that, "No matter how the uninsured are supported—whether by third-party payers, the presence of community health centers . . . or local government subsidies— we find no evidence that these efforts have the ability to eliminate, or even narrow, barriers to access to the extent that insurance can."[4]

Our nation needs to wake up and give all our people an equal opportunity to enjoy good health with dignity. In serving the uninsured, we clinicians who do this work appreciate what universal coverage would do to resolve this "great indignity." So many (but not all, of course) of our frustrations—and even more importantly, our patients' frustrations—would be resolved if America, like all other developed countries, adopted a system of universal coverage, such as national health insurance or an improved and expanded Medicare for All. Instead, we are headed in the direction of shifting more of the costs to the patients in the form of increased deductibles and co-pays.

The next two chapters further explore America's worship of the mantra (myth?) of "personal responsibility," our growing trend to "squeeze the patient," and how many religious groups in America, invoking the same mantra, have (surprisingly) failed to support universal coverage in America.

Summary of Key Points

- The "safety net" has an essential role in providing access to care for millions of Americans but is an extremely "piecemeal" solution.

- "Safety-net" care is often more rational care.

- "Safety-net" patients are often resentful and cynical about the way our nonsystem functions.

- People who use the "safety net" would have greatly increased access to the care they need if we had universal coverage.

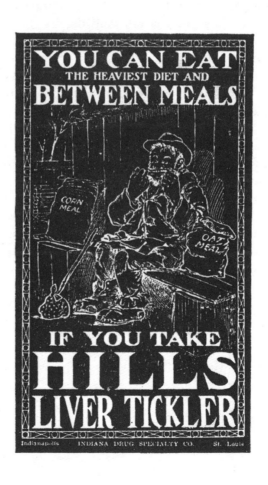

Chapter 6

Squeezing the Patient:
Co-Pays and Deductibles

Charlie Gomez is a 70-year-old man with high blood pressure and diabetes, both not well controlled because he fails to take his medicines correctly. Despite having Medicare, he does not come back for follow-up. He is ashamed that he owes us $52 and even more ashamed that he has no money for his co-payments. He winds up having a stroke for which he is briefly hospitalized. Luckily, it is not too severe, but it affects his short-term memory.

THERE IS A STRONG FEELING among many physicians and others in the business of American health care that everyone should personally share in the cost of their health care. Some even assert that people don't value what they don't pay for themselves. This philosophy ties in with the American creed of "personal responsibility," which is the philosophical antithesis of what conservatives term the "entitlement." Those with a more progressive or liberal bent talk in terms of human rights and justice instead of "entitlements," of health care being a human right, not a privilege. Language can define the parameters.

We're led to believe that rugged individualism—or is it really "everyone for himself"?—is the American way. And we hear much more about "personal responsibility" than we hear about our responsibilities as a society.

Idaho, the state where I live, is what could be termed a "bootstrap" state (as in, "pull yourselves up by your bootstraps"). A recent Idaho legislator suggested that the way a person could pay for health insurance would be "to go out and shoot an elk," sell the meat, and use the money to buy insurance. We could add this ingenious and original Idaho solution to the plethora of foundation-financed proposals for reducing the number of Americans without insurance.

Co-pays and deductibles perhaps in theory serve to reinforce the obligation to take an active role in one's own health care. This theory has major support from the insurance industry. But, in fact, the primary motivation behind the industry's support for co-pays and deductibles is financial:

1. Financial reason No.1: If the co-pays are substantial enough (say, $20 for a prescription or several hundred dollars for the Medicare inpatient deductible), they force the patient to share directly in a major portion of the cost of their health care. The expense to the insurer is thus diminished.

2. Financial reason No. 2: Co-pays and deductibles act as a barrier to care and reduce utilization. The net result is a cost savings (at least in the short run) to the insurance company. In all cases, to a greater or lesser degree, depending on the financial status of the person involved—the deductibles and co-pays discourage or limit utilization. While this saves money for the insurance companies, it can be terrible for the patient, especially if that patient is low-income and sick. Co-pays, as we have seen at our community health center (see Chapters 4 and 5), often lead people to delay or completely forgo needed care. Even for relatively well-to-do middle-class people, like many of the people I work with or myself, deductibles and co-pays are major incentives to delay care. How many of us have delayed preventive or other care because the financial disincentives have made us consider if the care was really necessary?

In an article that appeared in the *New England Journal of Medicine,* physician and economist Edie Rasell questioned the whole rationale underlying co-pays and deductibles.[1] She concluded that they failed to save money for the system. And

Canadian economist Robert Evans has noted that the effects of individual cost-savings are illusory if they do not save money for health care expenditures overall.[2] Indeed, the United States, with the highest rates of co-pays and deductibles of any of the developed countries, has by far the highest rate of spending for health care.

Why Do Physicians Support Co-Pays?

MANY PHYSICIANS SUPPORT the concept of co-pays as a tool to put the brakes on overutilization. However, it's not totally clear to me why physicians should be so concerned about what they consider to be overutilization, or what benefit they personally derive from limiting utilization in general. Are they lazy? Maybe they don't want to be bothered by problems they consider trivial. Maybe they don't like being awakened at 3 a.m. for those same trivial problems. Possibly they resent a certain attitude they sense from insured patients, especially from people with Medicaid, an attitude that seems to invoke the idea of "entitlement." I remember one local doctor who seemed quite offended when I talked about health care being a human right. "Does that mean that if they come to me for care, I can't refuse to take care of them?" he questioned angrily.

Some of the physicians' hard feelings about overutilization undoubtedly do come from experience. Nearly every physician in primary or emergency care has seen a Medicaid family where mom has brought in a child with the sniffles and then asks if the doctor can also examine the other two children because they too have stuffy noses. Or there are the drunks who stagger into the ER at 3 a.m. Somehow it doesn't seem right. The physician feels that if there had been a co-pay, mom wouldn't have brought her child in or asked to have the other children seen, or the drunk would have thought twice about the hour he picked to be seen. But is it fair to generalize from examples that seem to be "an abuse" of the system and advocate that there should be co-pays from everyone to discourage frivolous or unnecessary use? Of course, the Medicaid mom or the drunk may not have considered their use of services "frivolous." And I personally regard many of these alleged "frivolous" visits as opportunities to promote prevention, such as checking on immunizations and healthy lifestyles.

In their first draft outlining their plan for universal coverage, the American Academy of Family Physicians (AAFP) recognized the negative effects of co-pays and deductibles in causing people to delay or forgo needed care. In a break from the prevalent thinking in America about having the patient share costs, the AAFP in 2000 proposed a plan that offered universal coverage for primary care and preventive services without any co-pays or deductibles. They later modified the proposal to deliver only preventive and prenatal services without co-pays and to require a 20 percent co-pay on other primary care visits. They justified the change by invoking the "personal responsibility" paradigm that doctors and insurance companies are so fond of promoting. There is an inconsistency here, though it follows from the current conventional wisdom about payments for health care services. Are preventive services to be delivered without a co-payment because (1) they are so essential that the AAFP wants to be sure that people can afford them, or (2) the services are not valued enough by people who would forgo them rather than come up with a co-pay?

As for the argument that people don't value services they get for free, perhaps preventive services and immunizations should require co-payments too. That way, people would value those services more, right? On the other hand, those of us who regard primary care as prevention, especially for chronic diseases, would argue that co-pays are inappropriate and counterproductive to good health.

Co-Pays That Hurt

THEN THERE ARE THE co-pays that even well-insured people have to contend with in the case of serious illness. I recently saw a Hispanic couple in my clinic whose child had leukemia. They have health insurance coverage through his work, and their child is covered, but they cannot afford to pay the hefty 20 percent co-pay on their son's bills. What are their alternatives? Quit work so that their son can qualify for Medicaid or SCHIP? Spend less on groceries for the family? Personal bankruptcy is a strong option for the insured family with a tiny premature baby that runs up a $200,000 bill in the neonatal intensive care unit if the family is responsible for 20 percent of the bill, or $40,000. Interestingly enough, the AAFP proposal deals with this issue by including a catastrophic insurance component in their plan.

The problem lies in the payment system, not in the people who allegedly "abuse the system." The co-pay protects both the insurer and the provider of services from overuse. But what protects the patient, especially these days when the co-pays and deductibles are almost geometrically increasing? We have a growing number of patients with insurance who use our community health center because they can't afford their deductibles or co-pays. Some insurance plans now even require their members to pay up front for all drugs, meaning that they go without when they don't have the $50 or $120 in their pockets to shell out for an expensive medication.

There's no doubt that there should be improved patient education to promote more appropriate use of medical services. However, that educative process should deal with *both* under-utilization and overutilization. Unfortunately, co-pays and deductibles, being indiscriminate in their effect on utilization, often discourage *appropriate* care as well as inappropriate care. They are often a significant barrier for those people who have limited economic means despite having insurance coverage. The uninsured, who are responsible for full payment, have an even larger economic disincentive to use medical services. Overutilization is hardly a problem with the uninsured. In fact, the uninsured utilize medical services much less than the insured, even in a "safety-net" setting like a community health center. Studies show they utilize services at 60 percent of the rate of the insured.

There is ample evidence in the medical literature about the negative effects of co-pays on the health of low-income families. From the RAND Corporation study in 1986 to a recent study in the *Journal of the American Medical Association (JAMA)* showing an increase in bad outcomes when co-pays were instituted for drugs in Quebec,[3] studies demonstrate that co-pays lead to decreased utilization of necessary care and increased morbidity.

In the Quebec study, the institution of co-pays for drugs for the elderly led to a reduction in their use of essential drugs, an increase in serious adverse effects (hospitalization, long-term care admission or death), and a greater number of ER visits. I'm not aware of any scientific studies showing that co-pays lead to better health care outcomes, or evidence showing that higher co-pays lead to even better outcomes. Even in third-world countries, co-pays have been shown to have a negative effect upon health status.

The failure to use health care services when they are appropriately necessary leads to delayed care, a frequent situation with those who are uninsured. And now, we are increasingly seeing delayed care with the *under*insured, or those with high deductibles and co-pays. Delayed care means more serious illness and disability in the long run and higher costs. It costs much more to care for a serious illness. In addition, there are the human implications of unnecessary suffering, disability and death.

The "Safety Net" and Co-Pays

IN COMMUNITY AND MIGRANT health centers, which largely serve people who "fall between the cracks" for financial or geographical reasons, co-pays or "nominal fees" are nearly universal. The exceptions are people with Medicaid and those who qualify for "Health Care for the Homeless" programs. The federal bureau that oversees these clinics encourages these fees, partly to ensure the survival of the clinics, but perhaps also to reinforce the "personal responsibility" ethos. Maybe one of our missions is to "build character." However, in my experience, the higher the co-pays, the wider the cracks become for people to fall through. Obviously, these fees help support, sometimes in a major way, the operating budgets of these clinics. To some extent they are necessary so that the clinics can continue giving the services provided. Yet it has been very difficult for our clinics to sort out which patients are harmed by the policy. Many patients fail to come back for follow-up or don't get the medicines prescribed because, despite the low fees of these clinics, they cannot afford even minimal charges.

The Medicaid program generally has no co-pays. Where there are some minimal co-pays (such as for prescription drugs in a few states), they wind up costing more to administer than they produce in revenue. When the Medicaid program was established, the designers must have felt that poor people (for whom Medicaid was designed) did not have the resources to afford co-pays and deductibles. Although the lack of these payments is a sore point among many state legislators, it would be unrealistic to expect people with Medicaid to contribute any significant co-pay. Imposition of a co-pay would only lead to delayed or omitted care for the most vulnerable people, those who don't have the courage to challenge the system. People who have learned to manipulate the system will find ways to get around co-pays.

Nonetheless, there appears to be a movement in state legislatures to apply for waivers from the federal government (for example, under the new Health Insurance Flexibility and Accountability Demonstration Initiative, or HIFA) so they can impose co-pays on Medicaid patients. They're looking for ways to spend less, but I wonder if some of the motivation for the co-pays comes from a desire somehow to "punish" Medicaid recipients. To put the issue into perspective, would we favor, for example, charging co-pays for the many thousands of New Yorkers who enrolled in "disaster-relief Medicaid" after the September 11 disaster or for the unfortunate victims of Hurricane Katrina?

The Larger Picture

THE DILEMMA OF THE co-pays and deductibles has two poles. At one pole there is the specter of a plethora of unnecessary visits by people who have frivolous complaints (the "worried well"), such as we're told happens in countries like Germany and Japan. At the other pole, we have the American health care system, where those who cannot afford health care delay or just don't get the necessary care. And there are even many middle-class Americans who *can* afford health care but delay or skip their care anyway because of the co-pays and deductibles—an economic choice that may or may not be wise. It's likely that the European and

Japanese health systems may foster too much dependency on the part of patients, but in America, given the exorbitant cost of health care today, we may have gone too far in stressing *independence* as the standard. We are systematically encouraging or forcing people to delay or avoid care.

Looking at the larger picture (the overall health status of Americans and the cost of health care in America), co-pays and deductibles, as well as the large number of people without insurance, are undoubtedly contributing to our poor performance on both measures as compared to other countries. Why do we rank so poorly—mostly 20th or worse—on such measures as immunization rates, infant mortality, and life expectancy? Do our financial barriers to access mean that Americans delay care enough so that they eventually require more expensive specialists and hospital care, leading to more expensive procedures and cost overall?

If there were no co-pays or deductibles, we likely would have a subgroup of beneficiaries who would overuse the system, just as some people do with Medicaid today. But, given our American ethos of personal independence and self-reliance, it's doubtful the phenomenon of overuse would become very widespread. Besides, the great majority of Americans, with a few exceptions, do not enjoy spending the day sitting in the waiting rooms of clinics or emergency rooms. Our American health care system has been perversely skewed by a philosophy to "keep the patients out," a philosophy some medical residents pursued as if it were a badge of honor.

The transition of American health care toward for-profit HMOs, which benefit when patients don't come in for care, only served to reward the goal of "keeping the patients out." We need some balance. If we're committed to improving the "larger picture" referred to above (health status, total spending), and not just the "bottom line" of health care corporations, then at the very least we should do what we can to reduce the financial barriers to necessary care. And that means rethinking what we are doing with co-pays and deductibles. We also need to rethink how we deal with so-called "frivolous" complaints. Instead of creating financial barriers that discourage access to care we presume is "frivolous," we need to develop guidelines that can encourage care that is appropriate, cost-effective, and humane.

There used to be what was called "first dollar"[4] insurance, "in a distant land, long, long ago." How times have changed, at least for the non-Medicaid population. But what is the meaning of insurance after all? To insure against risks. What do co-pays and deductibles have to do with risk? The AAFP proposal places every American into one risk pool for primary care and prevention. Their plan is paid for through taxes, as opposed to insurance premiums, and it eliminates the co-pays and deductibles for certain—and in the original draft, *all*—primary care services. Conceptually, their original proposal could be looked at as having included (that is, paid for up front or prepaid) the co-pays and deductibles as an *integral part* of the coverage package. The original plan did away with these payments at the time of service for the express reason of eliminating the financial barriers that lead people to delay or altogether skip primary care visits and preventive services.

I don't think it's a good idea, but I wouldn't be opposed to charging co-pays or deductibles for people who could afford them—if it were really necessary for the financial survival of the system. I think it's a good idea to have co-pays for expensive brand-name medicines when a generic or over-the-counter inexpensive equivalent will do the job. And I agree with a *full* pay requirement for services that are not medically necessary. But so often we have difficulty figuring out who can and who cannot afford the co-pays. And even poor people, like Mr. Gomez, have pride and a desire to keep their dignity. Must we continue to turn away the people like Mr. Gomez—with all the attendant consequences, like a stroke—because of a philosophy ("personal responsibility") that no longer has a basis in reality? In today's America, given the high degree of poverty, the difficulty in making a living wage, and our expensive chaotic health system, "personal responsibility" has limited usefulness for almost anybody, let alone a person with limited resources like Mr. Gomez.

Any one of us could be wiped out financially with a serious illness or accident. We are all at risk. For those of us who are caregivers, think how badly we feel when we take care of a

person who has a personal disaster happen because of delayed
care, a delay that frequently occurs because that person feels that
she or he cannot afford the co-pay or minimal fee. It happens, and
we all know it. In my own practice, it happens on a daily basis.
As Harry and Louise speculated, "There must be a better way."

Summary of Key Points

- Co-pays and deductibles lead to an increase
  in delayed care or omitted care for everyone.

- Our high co-pays and deductibles likely
  contribute to our lower performance in key
  health status indicators compared to the other
  developed countries.

- Invoking "personal responsibility" to justify
  co-pays is a form of "blaming the victim."

- There is *no* scientific evidence to prove
  that higher co-pays lead to better health
  outcomes.

Chapter 7

Religion and Health Care Reform:
A Personal View

by C. Rocky White, MD

*"For I was hungry and you gave Me food; I was
thirsty and you gave Me something to drink; I was a
stranger and you brought Me together with yourselves
and welcomed and entertained and lodged Me;*

*I was naked and you clothed Me; I was sick and you
visited Me with help and ministering care; I was in
prison and you came to see Me."*

*Then the just and upright will answer Him, "Lord,
when did we see You hungry and gave You food, or
thirsty and gave You something to drink?*

*And when did we see You a stranger and welcomed
and entertained You, or naked and clothed You?*

*And when did we see You sick or in prison and came
to visit You?"*

*And the King will reply to them, "Truly, I tell you, in
as far as you did it to one of the least [in the estimation
of men] of these My brethren, you did it to Me."*

—Matthew 25:35-40, *Amplified Bible*

MANY CONSERVATIVE AMERICANS, particularly those who
espouse more fundamentalist religious beliefs, equate health care
reform with socialism, a concept they regard with disfavor. As
such, certain Christian groups have generally opposed universal
coverage solutions, such as national health insurance, that involve

a larger role for government. That's why so many religious groups in America have avoided taking real action toward promoting universal coverage despite the obvious humanitarian need.

The struggle for health care for all seems so consistent with what religious groups are supposed to be about. Here, in Matthew 25, Jesus tells the story of the final judgment in which the righteous are divided from the unrighteous and the criteria used to separate them. The question asked is painfully obvious— did you care for others?

There is no reference to a paradise inhabited by suicide bombers, Holy War or crusading soldiers, presidents, popes, talk show hosts, or pious weekly churchgoers.

Jesus said, "For I was hungry and you gave Me food; I was thirsty and you gave Me something to drink." Food and water? Yes! But so much more is meant by it. Nourishment for the body, mind, and spirit—including physical, emotional, mental, and spiritual well-being, security, peace, education, and the truth.

"I was a stranger (a foreigner, an illegal alien, a communist, a homosexual, a homeless skid row person, a person with a different viewpoint) and you brought Me together with yourselves and welcomed and entertained and lodged Me (treated me as one of your own)."

"I was naked (vulnerable, defenseless, poverty-stricken with no voice of my own to be heard on Capitol Hill) and you clothed Me (kept me warm, came to my defense, acted as my advocate, and embraced me with justice)."

"I was sick and you visited Me with help and ministering care (you provided me with health care!)."

"I was in prison (not just a cell with iron bars, but also a prison of mental illness; depression; sexual, verbal, and/or physical abuse; poverty; hopelessness and despair) and you came to see Me (you offered me hope and a chance)."

"Truly, I tell you, in as far as you did it to one of the least [in the estimation of men] of these My brethren (your fellow people, no matter who they are), you did it to Me."

Throughout American history, the impact of faith-based groups on politics is indisputable. References to God, Providence, and "all men being created equal" permeate nearly every aspect of our culture. In fact, most of the great social reformers—from Abe Lincoln, William Jennings Bryan, and Teddy Roosevelt to Martin Luther King Jr. spoke openly of their faith and spiritual convictions. As one historian speaking of Martin Luther King Jr., pointed out, "He led the charge of racial reform with a Bible in one hand and the Constitution in the other."

So why is it, then, that the "Moral Majority" or the "Christian Coalition" or the National Association of Evangelicals with its 30 million plus members has garnered so much political leverage and yet has been so ineffective in what most of its mainstream members feel to be the real issues that concern the message of Christ?

The Scriptures give us the impression that Jesus cared little for the political climate of his day during his earthly ministry. By his example, he taught the world that people, not power, is what interests God. Everyone, black or white, man or woman, rich or poor, is considered equal in God's eyes, and strength is not emitted from the barrel of a gun, but rests in kindness and compassion.

The history of how the Christian Right rose to its place of power within the Republican Party and the current political scene is beyond the scope of our discussion. But the reality of its influence is not. Throughout the past 30 years, faith-based groups have decided elections, influenced policy, and its leaders have had the ears of presidents. Yet, what have they accomplished?

As faith-based groups began to organize in the 1970s as a response to extremist secular and liberal ideology coming out of Washington, they initially focused their energies on three specific issues—mainly, the Supreme Court decisions to restrict school prayer, to limit the power of states to ban birth control, and to protect the right of women to abort a pregnancy. Later, the protection of free speech in the form of burning the American flag and the question of gay marriage would be added to the list. For the next 30 years, these so-called "wedge issues" would dominate the political climate of the Religious Right and the Republican Party and would eventually lead to 6 years of Republican domination in Washington under the George W. Bush administration.

These well-intentioned, faith-based groups became the pillars of power in an administration that funneled the funds of the federal treasury to the richest in the land; created a prescription drug plan for seniors that all but guaranteed the continued profit frenzy of the pharmaceutical industry; tore holes in social safety nets with budget reductions in order to maintain tax cuts for the wealthy; and ignored the need for health care reform.

And through it all, where was the church?

The truth is the road to hell is paved with good intentions. Despite 6 years of conservative Republican domination in Washington, this country is no closer to a ban on abortion or flag burning or the reinstatement of school prayer than it was when Ronald Reagan made them a platform promise in 1980.

Well-meaning people of faith have been duped. These wedge issues, when spun correctly by the Republican power brokers, have been able to evoke fear and stir deep emotions. But the beauty of these wedge issues lies in the fact that they win elections and cost nothing!

Banning abortion, flag burning, or gay marriage, or reinstating school prayer doesn't cost us anything! You don't have to raise taxes, you can sleep with your conscience clear, and you don't have to make any personal sacrifice.

So what does all this have to do with the role of faith-based groups in the world of politics and health care reform?

First, we have to ask ourselves if the church should be involved in politics at all. In Luke 20, Jesus was asked if it was right for believers to pay taxes to a Caesar who considered himself to be a god. Christ held up a Roman coin with a likeness of Caesar embossed upon it and replied, "Render to Caesar the things that are Caesar's, and to God the things that are God's." Although the vision that Christ had was of a spiritual salvation and a "Heavenly Kingdom," his immediate ministry was natural and earthly, and he recognized that we as humans are still part of this natural world, and we have natural governments and laws.

Before his ascension, Jesus gave the command to the church to "go into all the world and preach the Gospel" (the Good News of a God who cares about people). And in Matthew 5, Jesus told his followers that they are the "salt of the earth." Salt was used as a preservative in the days before refrigeration to keep food from spoiling and decay. It is here that Jesus implies that people of faith who recognize a concerned and loving God are to be dispersed throughout society, preserving it from the decay and rottenness of greed, oppression, and violence.

Jesus also taught that you will know a tree by the fruit it bears (Matthew 7:20). And the Apostle Paul, writing in Galatians 5:22-23, pointed out that "The fruit of the (Holy) Spirit [the work which His presence within accomplishes]—is love, joy (gladness), peace, patience (an even temper, forbearance), kindness, goodness (benevolence), faithfulness (meekness, humility), gentleness, self-control (self-restraint, continence)."

Here in the United States, our current form of government makes every attempt to prevent the state from influencing religion with the same fervor as it does to prevent organized religion from controlling government. However, that does not mean that religious ideas or people of faith cannot or should not be involved in the political process.

In fact, from the previous Scriptures quoted, Jesus tells his followers to "bear fruit and be salt" in an evil and decaying world.

We see in Matthew 25 that the mission of the church is about love, compassion, and putting people first. And healing and providing health care is part of that commission.

Throughout history, religious organizations of all faiths have been at the forefront of reaching out to the sick and poor through charity hospitals, soup kitchens, homeless shelters, etc. Yet, despite these efforts, hundreds of thousands are still homeless, millions go to bed hungry every night, and tens of millions have no effective access to health care. And that is just here in the United States.

The truth is, even the most powerful and wealthiest religious organizations in the world have been ineffective in combating poverty and poor health. Part of the reason, as we have discussed, is that religious groups have used their influence to push for issues that have little or nothing to do with God's commission. Yes, we have a few selfless, dedicated individuals doing what they can in remote rural and inner city clinics and shelters, and they do touch many lives. But in the scheme of things, they may as well be draining the ocean with a 5-gallon bucket.

Poverty and, to maintain the focus of this book, adequate access to health care is part of the great commission of faith. And in our culture—because we have chosen a constitutional, democratically controlled republic, separate from the power of organized religion—the only avenue we have to effect and implement major social reform is through the halls of government. Only the federal government has the jurisdiction and the means to make the kind of changes necessary to provide adequate access to health care for all of its citizens.

The modern church in this nation does not have the cohesiveness, the legislative power, or the financial leverage to effect the changes needed to fight the war on poverty or to bring about health care reform. Our open system of government, however, which mandates separation of state from the direct influence of organized religion, does have mechanisms of influence through the process of elected representation. And the church, like any other lobby—religious or secular—should use them.

Some of the great social reforms of American history are products of a faith-based message from those who understood how to strike the balance. Abolition, child labor protections, civil service and election reform, women's right to vote, labor's right to strike, civil rights and voting rights, electing U.S. Senators by popular vote, and even protecting savings accounts by the establishment of the FDIC—all came through forceful characters who "held a Bible in one hand and the Constitution in the other."

The struggles for these reforms were vetted against insurmountable odds and came with a price of personal sacrifice. Teddy Roosevelt (although not the Bible thumper that William Jennings Bryan was), in his quest for civil service reform and bringing down the power of the Tammany Hall political machines, nearly trashed his own political career in the process. For William Jennings Bryan, it did cost him his political career. For Martin Luther King Jr., it cost him his life!

But the difference between the wedge issue rhetoric of today's modern church and the faith-based reformers of the nineteenth and twentieth centuries lies in the outcomes. The social reforms of the last two centuries made a difference in people's lives and exemplified the message of a loving God, as Jesus taught in Matthew 25.

So to say that faith and religious groups have no place in the American political scene is to expose one's ignorance of history. We make every attempt (and I would say, rightfully so) to separate the direct political process from the power of organized religion through various steps and limitations. But we should not and, in fact, cannot discount the contribution that religious groups can make in acting as a moral compass for our elected leaders, especially if they act as advocates for changes that actually would make a difference in people's lives—such as fighting for universal access to health care. This would truly be a pro-life message.

But what about the secular view of politics and reform? It seems that, over the last 30 years, conservative religious groups have drifted into the ranks of the Republican Party primarily out of a perceived need for survival. Many faith-based groups, and even many progressive-minded women who have made the choice to forgo a career and become "stay-at-home moms," have been castigated and feel there is no place for them within the ranks of the Democratic Party. It seems a shame that a party that has embraced platform ideals of social conscience, equality, and environmental awareness would hold so passionately to its secular ideals that it has alienated itself from mainstream America and especially many faith-based groups. In the quest to draw large lines of distinction in the separation of church and state, many extremists on the left have pushed that agenda to create a separation of faith from society.

It is perfectly understandable why faith-based groups would recoil into a striking position when elements of the extreme left (which are just as much a problem as the extreme right) create their own wedge issues of abortion, gay rights, or removing religious icons from sight, whether public or private. After the 2006 mid-term elections, the Republicans learned that religious conservatives are fed up with their smoke-and-mirrors. The Democrats must recognize that moderate people of faith are interested in a platform of social reform and, if they are going to be successful, they are going to have to moderate their own extremists and embrace an attitude of "religious tolerance."

According to *American Piety in the 21st Century*, the Baylor Religion Survey (September 2006), 95 percent of Americans believe in a "higher power" and 84 percent regard themselves as Christian. Although only about 5 percent of Americans represent other religions, such as Jewish, Muslim, Buddhist, etc., their views of a concerned God and social justice need to be taken into account as well. People of faith represent a huge chunk of the electorate that neither party can afford to ignore.

So, how does one build a coalition for a platform of social awareness without compromising deep convictions?

First, we must be aware that politics is a game of compromise; faith is not. Each of us has a limit. Each of us will only bend so far in our own personal convictions. Consider poor old Tevye, the main character in the musical "Fiddler on the Roof." Three times his values were challenged with the marriage of his three oldest daughters. The first daughter challenged his social values by marrying the man she loved, not the man her father arranged for her—tradition! The second daughter challenged his political views and married a Bolshevik—tradition! Both times Tevye (despite tradition) relented and blessed their marriages. But the third daughter married a Christian, and Tevye, a Jew, turned his back on her. He could bend socially and politically, but he could not compromise his faith!

Imagine that! A musical with an object lesson! And one we should all take to heart. Faith is a powerful motivating factor—it causes people to hate so much that they are willing to fly a jet into a building and kill thousands, or to love so much that they would allow themselves to be crucified for the sake of others. Thankfully, our founding fathers had enough foresight to see that because there are so many differing views of faith and that allowing one of those views to dominate politically can end up being injurious, they created a government that is insulated from organized religion. But you still cannot remove the effects of faith from the process anymore than we can remove the secular and humanistic views of the world. This is the government we have chosen, and this is the process we need to accept.

So, how do we get beyond our irreconcilable grievances and start making a difference? We must recognize that some issues will never be resolved. I doubt that I will ever live to see the day that the Catholic Church reaches a compromise on abortion with the National Organization of Women. Even if the Moral Majority managed to elect an administration that stacked the deck on the Supreme Court and overturned Roe vs. Wade, there is just as good a chance that the next generation will load the Court back to the left, and on and on it will go. But we can still effect social reform if we don't allow our pride to get in the way, damaging the opportunities we have for meaningful reform on issues we can do something about.

The move, therefore, to an effective social agenda (in this case, health care reform) lies not in compromise, but in finding the common ground and striving for the common good. A secular view of reform that sees the need to transform health care based on the intrinsic liberal ideals of human rights as a natural extension of social evolution should in no way conflict with the same ideals simply because they were expressed by a religious leader. At the same time, business can also find the common ground, realizing that its very existence depends upon a healthy workforce and an affordable means to maintain it.

This book is exhaustive in its portrayal of a health care system that is wasteful, inefficient, unjust, and collapsing under its own weight. Not only is reform needed to provide a social safety net to the poor and those who have no voice—in effect, extending human rights or fulfilling the commands of a loving God—but it is imperative to preserving the social fabric of the middle class. As we have demonstrated, even business—both large and small—is losing its ability to compete in an ever-shrinking global economy.

In conclusion, it is evident that secular liberals, religious fundamentalists, and business have a common ground in the fight to reform the health care system. And we have demonstrated that a single-payer system that is publicly financed and accountable to the people is the only mechanism that meets the demands of social justice with the application of sound business principles.

MORALITY QUIZ:

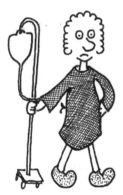

ALLOWING 40+ MILLION PEOPLE TO GO WITHOUT DECENT ACCESS TO HEALTH CARE IN THE RICHEST COUNTRY IN THE WORLD IS (CHOOSE ONE):

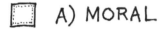 A) MORAL

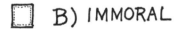 B) IMMORAL

© 2002 by Bob LeBow

Chapter 8

Public Health:
We're All on This Planet Together

Juan Rivera is a 54-year-old uninsured farmworker who was hospitalized with fever, weight loss, and an abnormal chest X-ray. His skin test and other tests are negative for tuberculosis, and he recovers enough to be discharged from the hospital. He was to follow up with a lung specialist for further evaluation, but when he gets to the specialist's office, he is asked for $100 up front before he can be seen. Discouraged with the system, he gives up and decides to forgo medical care. He shows up at our clinic several months later having lost another 40 pounds. His sputum smear now shows sheets of acid-fast bacilli (tuberculosis).

FOR THE SHORTSIGHTED who put faith in the mantra of "personal responsibility," there is a failure to realize that, when it comes to the spread of infectious diseases, lack of access to care can lead to public health catastrophes. In reality, we're all on this planet together.

Fortunately, Juan Rivera's tuberculosis turned out not to be a multiple-drug-resistant strain, but he did manage to infect at least one other person in his household, and perhaps others. Maybe our clinic could have done more to follow up on Juan, to make sure that he came back for care. We could have helped lead him through a maze of paperwork and bureaucracy that might have qualified him for some kind of medical assistance. In fact, because of people like Juan, we applied for (and received) grant funds to hire an extra social worker. That's what we need to help solve access-to-care dilemmas for all the Juans who need similar help in negotiating America's hodgepodge of a health care system.

In the past, when there were infectious disease problems, public health departments—at least where I was working—used to have adequate staffing to do epidemiological work-ups. They could both investigate contacts and follow up on people who fell between the cracks. Not so anymore. Budget and staffing cuts have severely restricted public health capabilities in America.[1] Of course, in Juan's case, we didn't even know at first that he had tuberculosis, and maybe he didn't have the disease when he first came in. It's often an elusive illness to diagnose. But his lack of the means to pay for care—and his frustration and shame at being drubbed by the system—led him to give up even trying to gain access to care.

America has thousands of Juan Riveras, thousands of people who are on the street spreading their diseases to other people. Some of them are recent immigrants who have unrecognized and untreated infectious diseases. They may have multiple-drug-resistant tuberculosis, like the California schoolgirl who infected several of her classmates. Or they may have HIV/AIDS, hepatitis, chlamydia, syphilis, or infectious skin diseases. They may be avoiding care because they are afraid of what they might have, but more often they avoid or delay care because they can't afford it.

The paradoxical and ironic twist to this dilemma is that we all pay for the care in the long run. As Juan's case illustrates, once these people have a catastrophic event and gain entry to our system, they get the specialty care and the expensive diagnostic tests they need. Unfortunately, their care is often much more expensive because they delayed the care in the first place or had problems gaining timely access to our system. Juan wound up spending about 6 months at a rehabilitation hospital and eventually recovered—and somebody paid the bills. I suspect it would have been more cost-effective (and humanitarian and decent) to have made sure that Juan had received more timely care. Beyond Juan's personal suffering, one also has to consider the public health implications.

Public Health and Chronic Disease

TIMELY CARE HAS A public health impact beyond infectious diseases. In the area of chronic disease, such as diabetes and hypertension, delayed care has many adverse effects with public health implications; for example:

- A higher rate of complications.

- Increased mortality and morbidity (as from heart attacks, strokes, limb amputations, blindness, kidney failure).

- Increased overall costs.

- More disability.

- A greatly increased level of human suffering.

Trying to quantify exactly how much we actually spend in excess each year because of delayed care is very difficult to do. The various methods used to extract that data can be "massaged and manipulated" to support many opinions. Although any set of data can be challenged, I have found the book *Inside the American Healthcare Crisis* by Balcar and Mueller to be an intriguing and very sophisticated attempt to quantify the cost of what they call "care denial-induced illness."[2] According to the authors (even using data from 1998), the overall cost to the system resulting from denied or delayed care from the uninsured or poorly insured exceeds $200 billion a year! That's an additional $600 a year in increased health care cost for every man, woman, and child in this country!

The inadequate treatment of chronic disease takes an overwhelming psychological and financial toll upon families, not to mention the cost to society as a whole. On an individual basis, consider the financial, and human, implications of a 60-year-old previously healthy man who has a debilitating stroke that might have been prevented with adequate care. Perhaps this man's misfortune helps a whole industry devoted to home care, rehabilitation, and durable medical equipment. But the human costs for this heretofore active, productive person—and the wife who must now cut back on her active life to care for him—are daunting, to say the least. Multiply this type of situation by a few million and we have a public health problem of the highest magnitude as well as a problem with significant impact upon our nation's economy.

America has recognized the public health importance of treating certain conditions. We have taken a patchwork (or categorical), as opposed to comprehensive, approach to address some specific problems; for example, HIV/AIDS coverage through Ryan White funds, prenatal care through expansion of Medicaid income criteria, or family planning through Title X funding. There used to be more local health department involvement in infectious diseases, such as follow-up for tuberculosis and venereal diseases, but resources have been stretched to a point where these activities are often impossible to carry out.

Access to care in a more comprehensive sense has public health implications. As such, there has been some recognition of the merits of population-based approaches to providing access to care. One good example is the State Children's Health Insurance Program (SCHIP), which has provided expansion of health insurance coverage for children since it was enacted in 1997. Sadly, though, according to the most recent data released by the Campaign for Children's Health Care, as of the summer of 2006, 9 million children under age 18 still have no health care coverage, and most of those kids are in working families![3] Years ago, we recognized that low-income people and seniors needed help getting health care. As a result, we implemented or supported Medicaid, Medicare, and a variety of "safety nets" such as Community and Migrant Health Centers and public hospitals. All of these approaches, for one reason or another, are either incomplete or inadequate. And these "solutions" have created a system that is at once unwieldy, overly complicated, duplicative, expensive, and grossly inequitable.

The New Twist to Wake Us Up: Bioterrorism

NOW WE HAVE A new twist with a public health dimension that further brings into question the validity of the old mantra about "personal responsibility": bioterrorism. Should Americans be expected to fend for themselves when they come down with—or think they may have—anthrax, enteric diseases from a poisoned water supply, neurological damage from poison gas, or even worse, smallpox? Will each person so affected be expected to show her/his health insurance card at the front desk and/or be expected to foot the bill, no matter what? "Sorry, you've got a $2,000 deductible, and you'll have to come up with $100 up front before the doctor will see you with that blistering rash covering your whole body."

I suspect that, using typical American ingenuity, we will come up with a special fund, perhaps the "Anthrax, Bioterrorism, and Chemical Disabilities (ABCD)" Fund. The fund will have, of course, appropriately complicated screening and eligibility criteria. And it will pay for services related to the War on Terrorism—assuming that other insurances are billed first, of course.

The whole emerging issue of the health effects of bioterrorism does bring into focus the craziness of our current system for financing health care. We are forced to look at how we are all in this together. We are a community, a society, and what some of us do affects everyone else. Terrorist retaliation for what we as a nation might do in Afghanistan, Palestine, Iraq, or anywhere else in the world can cause death and disability for those Americans who are unfortunate enough, like the people in the World Trade Center, to be in the wrong place at the wrong time. Obviously, the same dependence on chance and luck applies to accidents.

And a similar situation applies to a great degree, though not totally, to chronic diseases. Many of these ailments are more than likely to be caused, at least somewhat, by environmental factors and/or our genetic inheritance. It makes no sense, either financial or humanitarian, to continue our current way of covering health care in America. Our system is looking increasingly like a combination of two TV shows: "Wheel of Fortune" and "Survivor." Don't get sick. And you'd better not be sipping your espresso at a café when a suicide bomber walks in and lights his or her match.

In the past two decades, as the emphasis in health care in America has shifted away from "care" and the patient to "cost" and business, the role of public health has diminished. In implementing a steady rise in our co-pays and deductibles, the system has ignored the public health consequences of delayed care, most notably for infectious diseases and chronic illnesses. With respect to chronic diseases, the victims have largely been people of limited means. In contrast, the infectious disease threat (as with anthrax, Lyme disease, or multiple-drug-resistant tuberculosis) does not select out any particular economic class. In trying to discourage so-called "overutilization" (see Chapter 2, "the Monster We Have Created"), we have encouraged an ambiance of underutilization, a much more serious problem with serious public health consequences.

Public health deals with population groups, but it also deals with each individual. Sometimes the two objects of public health efforts appear to come into conflict, such as when WHO policy dictated when people should *not* be treated for tuberculosis—for fear of creating drug resistance and untreatable disease. And the same international debate is beginning for HIV/AIDS. The situation in the third world is, of course, different from ours. But, if America had universal coverage, our own "third-world" population would be largely freed from the ethical dilemma of defining public versus individual needs.

Meanwhile, we're all at risk as long as we perpetuate a system that seems to be designed to ignore public health considerations, factors that have been assumed (incorrectly) to be of minor financial importance and not a positive force for the short-term bottom line. It's as if some of us (maybe the CEOs and executives of the insurance companies) are not on this world with the rest of us. Maybe when we accept the premise that "we're all on this planet together," and that—rich or poor, whites or people of color—we're all susceptible to the same public health (and other health) risks, we'll understand better why our health care system needs fundamental change.

In the United States, we do have a successful example, at least from the perspective of the patient, of a systems approach to health care coverage that places some of us (those 65 and over) "on the same planet" with regard to health care. It uses a "one risk pool" mechanism, and it's called Medicare. Unfortunately, it's under attack despite its popularity among our seniors.

Summary of Key Points

- Everyone in America has a shared risk for infectious disease, terrorist attacks, and (to some degree) chronic illnesses.

- From a public health viewpoint, it is only just that the whole community share the financial risk associated with these events or conditions.

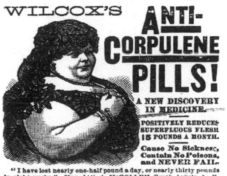

Chapter 9

Blaming the Victim:
A Bad Rap for Medicare

*"Whatever the solution is, we don't want more
government. Anything but big government."*
—A small business owner in Idaho

*"I don't want the government messing with my
Medicare."*
—An elderly Florida man, 1994

IN THE AMERICAN WEST, where many people—health care
providers and patients alike—have an almost innate distrust of
government, it is difficult to sell the concept of Medicare for All.
Physicians are especially wary and incredulous, especially since
Medicare began to crack down on billing irregularities in a manner that doctors perceived to be arbitrary and heavy-handed.
When Medicare cut its reimbursement to doctors by 5.4 percent
at the beginning of 2002, all because of a flawed formula based
on the GDP, physicians became even more dissatisfied. Hospital
administrators have also been extremely frustrated with
Medicare's onerous regulations as well as alleged underpayments. As for the beneficiaries, although they are often confused
by the workings of Medicare, they appreciate the "safety net" that
the program provides for them, even if it is incomplete. And seniors fiercely defend "their Medicare."

When asked how much overhead Medicare has, it's amazing
how providers and patients alike come up with grossly inflated
estimates. A gynecologist colleague of mine guessed, "It must be
70 percent." And I've had seniors in a polled audience figure that it

had to be at least 50 percent. They assume that since the federal government runs Medicare, it has to be wasteful. They believe the myth that the private sector is always better, more efficient, than the government. Never mind that over 95 cents of every Medicare dollar is spent on health care, compared to an average of 85 cents (and, in some cases, as little as 76 cents in the private sector. (See Chapter 1, Myth #4, for more discussion.) Remind us again, why is it so important to keep financing of health care in the private sector?

Part of Medicare's efficiency comes from its sheer size, an advantage that would be replicable if we had national health insurance. Other factors also contribute to its low overhead, such as: no profit motive, no middlemen or commissions, no onerous eligibility requirements, simplified forms, and no need to market a product. On the other hand, many providers, especially hospitals, complain that the regulatory burden of Medicare raises their administrative costs.

However, in the past two decades, Medicare has not been alone in causing added administrative headaches for providers. Especially for physicians, but also for hospitals and other types of providers, Medicare's rules and restraints have often been a lesser evil than the dictates of the managed-care industry. Even with regard to reimbursement, despite the complaints about Medicare, managed-care plans have often paid providers even less.

The Medicare model offers great opportunities for savings in administrative costs. As mentioned above, overall administrative costs in the United States consume an estimated 25 to 30 percent of health care spending. Canada's single-payer system spends less than half that percentage on administrative costs. Even if all we did was cut our administrative cost in half, this country would save more than $300 billion a year (based on 2006 spending), money that could be spent on patient care and prevention instead of marketing, duplication of services, paperwork, profits, commissions, and astronomical CEO salaries. These administrative savings alone could easily allow us to afford universal coverage in America. Imagine the further savings if we went to a system like Medicare with an overhead of only 5 percent or less!

Yet there is distrust of the government, a gut feeling—though unsubstantiated by hard figures—that the government (Medicare and Medicaid) is less efficient than the private sector.

Medicare as the Victim

From the patient (or consumer) point of view, Medicare's shortcoming is that it's an incomplete program, not comprehensive enough. In a feature article on Medicare reform that appeared in *The New York Times* in the summer of 2000,[1] the Baltimore seniors who were interviewed agreed upon a simple message. They didn't want Medicare "reformed" or privatized. "Improve and expand it," they advised. But it's a different story from the provider side, which all too often feels put out and irritated by Medicare. It didn't used to be that way. In the "good old days" when Medicare started, over the objections of the AMA, it simply paid the bills that were submitted. What a deal. Of course, the "blank check" days had to end. Too many providers—and others who were just out to defraud the system without even providing a service—learned how to bill Medicare so as to maximize their income (see Chapter 2).

Even after Medicare began to put some restraints on the system, such as Diagnosis Related Groups (DRGs), providers figured out how to maximize their reimbursement by such practices as "unbundling" or "up-coding." America's largest for-profit hospital chain, HCA/Columbia, paid a first installment $745 million fine in 2001 for the fraudulent billing of Medicare, largely related to "up-coding," or coding illnesses at a higher rate of severity than merited. Medicare, and Medicaid too, were being, and continue to be, ripped off, and then blamed for being too bureaucratic.

Congress became aware of some of the abuses and attempted to put more controls on the health care industry in the Balanced Budget Amendment of 1997. Unfortunately, their action did "throw some of the babies out with the bath water." America's "free-enterprise" ethic combined with the entrepreneurial spirit of medical providers may have contributed to the problem. Adding to the dilemma were others who were out-and-out crooks doing blatant fraud. Some of the worst abuses came from home health agencies, nursing homes, so-called "Medicaid mills," and for-profit hospitals. But the billing abuse has been more generalized. My former nurse, checking over the bill that was sent to Medicare by the Pennsylvania hospital where she had had a pacemaker implanted, noted that Medicare had been billed for two pacemakers—at $4,000 each. A billing error? I wonder how many of these billing errors have been omissions (undercharges) rather than overcharges. I'd bet not as many.

With the ongoing losses of tax monies that have been incurred by Medicare and Medicaid, Congress and the Health Care Financing Administration (HCFA, now CMS, the Centers for Medicare & Medicaid Services) had the obligation to take some action. When it came out in the press in 2000 that Medicare had paid out $23 billion for billings that were not warranted, the story was presented in such a way as to criticize Medicare. Yet a grossly understaffed HCFA (or CMS)—it still has only about 4,600 employees to oversee a program that pays out nearly $500 billion a year—did not have the resources to police such a huge nationwide program. Attacked by both sides—by the providers for having too many regulations and not reimbursing enough, and by Congress for reimbursing too much and not regulating enough—Medicare has come to be an example of "blaming the victim." Someone had to overbill or file fraudulent claims, thus ripping off Medicare and the American people. Those are the people who should be blamed, not Medicare.

Unfortunately, recent high-handed tactics by Medicare—with unfair, even draconian legal and financial mandates—have embittered many providers. Combined with low reimbursement, these actions have led many physicians to stop seeing Medicare patients. Medicare is moving to change how it deals with physicians, to modify the high-handedness. Some limited legislation to improve the situation passed the House in December 2001, and more substantial legislative relief is being debated in Congress. Changes involving public policy often come slowly, as with most governmental actions. They require debate in a public arena, a disadvantage *and* advantage of a public (versus private) system.

With the events of September 11, the public seems to have retreated a bit from the knee-jerk feeling that the private sector is always better than the public—or government—sector. At least with public safety, as with airport security, defense, police, and fire protection, the American public (and Congress, which voted for it) supports government solutions. Health care, like transportation, defense, and education, is an issue of vital public interest and safety (viz, the anthrax and smallpox threats). And good health is in the economic interest of the nation, not just the responsibility of each individual.

Expanding and Improving Medicare

MEDICARE WAS DESIGNED FOR 1965, and health care in twenty-first-century America has little resemblance to what it was then. Medicare needs to be improved and expanded. A concise summary explaining how this transformation could be accomplished is presented in a March 2001 "think piece" from the Economic Policy Institute.[2] However, powerful lobbies in this nation are working hard to prevent the kind of changes needed to make a real difference. These special interests (which, sadly, have garnered the support of the American Medical Association) strive intensely to maintain the status quo. Such is the case of the pharmaceutical industry and the recent Medicare Part D legislation. Congress had before it the golden opportunity to provide relief to our seniors for the ever-growing burden of prescription medication costs in an atmosphere of fairness and cost containment. Instead (with the multimillion-dollar influence of the pharmaceutical and for-profit insurance industry lobby), our system of privatized fragmentation was expanded into an even more convoluted and confusing program that even the most astute medical experts had a hard time assimilating. This program made it illegal for the government to contract with drug manufacturers and buy prescriptions in bulk. Never mind that the federal government already does that through the Veterans Administration and has saved our veterans and the taxpayers literally hundreds of millions of dollars. Instead, it handed the capacity to buy in bulk and then tack on a margin of profit and administrative fees to such giants as Humana and UnitedHealth Group, which together control 45 percent of the Medicare D prescription drug plans and 33 percent of the managed Medicare market—all at taxpayer expense! Then, to add insult to injury, the Bush administration managed to conceal the true cost of this program from Congress until it was passed into law. The actual cost of the Medicare D prescription plan over 10 years will be tens of billions of dollars in excess of original estimates. And the purpose of all this? To funnel taxpayer money that was meant to provide health care to our seniors back to Wall Street, and to starve Medicare financially so that reforming it will require its privatization.

Such is the strategy that has been used in other countries, such as Canada and the United Kingdom, when conservative governments have tried to favor the private sector. The Bush administration could have been more aggressive in its efforts to roll back the 5.4 percent reduction in Medicare physician payments that occurred at the beginning of 2002 as a result of a faulty bureaucratic formula. And President Bush's projected budget allocations for Medicare (put out in March 2002) were woefully inadequate. As Paul Krugman noted in an op-ed piece in *The New York Times*, ". . . We have already reached the point at which we must either come up with more money or deny care to retirees. . . . Medicare payments have already been squeezed beyond their limits, to the point where recipients can't find doctors willing to take them. Something will have to give, and soon."[3]

"Blaming the victim" (Medicare) plays to the interests of corporate America and enlists the support of an anti-government public bias that has been cultivated and nurtured by corporate and certain other political interests over the past two decades. Yet Medicare has demonstrated—at least for every American 65 years old and older—the feasibility of an equitable, theoretically affordable, and universal "safety net" for health care in America. There are very few seniors who would advocate for dismantling Medicare. So it's time Americans woke up, stopped "blaming the victim," and started protecting their safety net from those who would destroy it and leave those who are economically disadvantaged with second- or third-rate health care.

Americans could also start learning from the "Medicares," or national health insurance systems, of other countries, though many Americans seem to have an innate distrust of anything "foreign."

Summary of Key Points

- Medicare needs to be improved and expanded, not privatized or dismantled.

- National health insurance, with "one risk pool" for all Americans, similar to (an improved) Medicare, is *not* socialized medicine.

- "The government" is *not* an alien force. It is us.

Chapter 10

We Don't Want a Health Care System
Like They Have in Those Foreign Countries

"We have a health system that is the pride of the world."
—Professor David B. Williams[1]

*"We're different from the other countries. I've heard
say you're just a number there."*
—A 65-year-old female patient

MY WORK IN HEALTH CARE has taken me to 21 foreign countries,
nearly all in the third world. I've also worked in Russia, which
used to be categorized as "second world" but now might be better described as "otherworldly," at least with respect to its health
care system. I've learned something about the health systems in
other Western countries, especially Canada. I don't dare claim to
be an expert on the European systems. However, I was once
conned into giving a lunch presentation on the Scandinavian
health systems at a meeting of Physicians for a National Health
Program (PNHP). I partially prepared for that talk by using a network of friends to get feedback via the Internet from Denmark
and Norway.

Each developed country has its own unique system with its
particular advantages and disadvantages. No system is perfect,
and all of them are either currently experiencing financial problems or have had them recently. All are affected by politics. All
have their critics and their defenders. And none of them are static.
They all have been changing to reflect changing needs and
changing economies. Some countries have experimented with
privatization, usually under the aegis of conservative governments. So far, privatization has found a niche in several countries,

but the trend has shifted back toward the strengthening of publicly funded services.

Every developed country—with the exception of the United
States—has made a genuine effort to assure that every person living in that country has health care coverage (not just access).
And, by and large, they have succeeded. No one in those countries has to worry about going without needed health care. It's
true they may have to wait if the care is not urgent. In some cases,
as in end-of-life situations, they may not receive heroic measures.
But no one in those other countries has to worry about declaring
bankruptcy because of their health care bills.

Even in the third world, where I have worked at a systems
level for nearly 30 years, most countries recognize health care as
a human right. Their constitutions include a right to health care.
They have national public health systems, which act as a safety
net for even the poorest people. Unfortunately, their ability to
staff and supply their health care systems is often minimal.

The United States stands almost alone in the world in its failure to recognize health care as a human right. Instead we consider
health care as an economic commodity. If you can afford it,
you can get it. If not, you're out of luck—despite the myth that
"anyone can go to the emergency room for care." Unfortunately,
America is now exporting its market-driven philosophy of health
care to other countries.[2] The effects could be disastrous for poor
people in some of those countries, especially those in Latin
America.

Considering that market-driven health care has been such a
failure here, it's ironic, and sad, that we are selling our approach
abroad. American corporations are trying to make profits abroad
by encouraging the privatization of the parts of health sectors that
offer potential for profit. Creating HMOs for the well-to-do.
Diverting social security funds to private enterprise. The poor
will be lucky to get the leftovers. And opposition to our "health
care imperialism" may be stifled by trade agreements. The net
results will likely be the raiding of social security funds in these
countries and the further marginalization of the poor and their
ability to get access to health care. In fact, the Bush administration has even tried to coerce other countries into lifting their price

controls on such things as prescription medications. Besides profit, I suppose part of their motivation is so that we don't look so bad.

Americans Are Clueless
on What Happens in Other Countries

AMERICANS ARE GENERALLY UNINFORMED about what is happening in other countries with respect to health care. They have no idea that corporate America is actively exporting our profit-driven approach to both industrialized and developing countries around the world. And they are unaware that all the other industrialized countries spend much less than the United States on health care and yet cover all their people. They don't know that:

1. If you took the top 10 most expensive health care systems in the world outside the United States, their average per capita spending is just over $3,700 per year. Compare this to the United States at $5,711.[3]

2. Calculated as a percentage of Gross Domestic Product (GDP), U.S. health care spending is now 15.2 percent of its GDP compared to the next most expensive country, Switzerland, at 11.5 percent.

3. Put another way, we spend 35 percent more per capita and about 40 percent more than the average GDP of the other top 10 most expensive health care systems in the world. Despite this, we still have 46 million citizens who are uninsured, and we have some of the worst health outcome indicators of all the industrialized nations! (Note: By the time this book goes to press (in 2007), per capita spending will exceed $7,000, and we will have already surpassed 16 percent of GDP.)

Our excess expenditures for health care are despite—or maybe partly *because of*—our failure to cover 15 percent of our people. Indeed, Donald Light argues that universal access to health care would greatly lower the overall cost of health care in the United States. It would grossly simplify our current complex systems for billing, marketing, and administration—and save money. In an article entitled "Health Care for All: A Conservative Case," Light points out that our overhead (about 25 percent) is about three times that spent in countries "with private care but universal access, such as Germany, Japan, and The Netherlands."[4]

The American public has pretty much bought into the myths about foreign health care. These myths have been carefully nurtured and financed by the special interests. The ingrained myths include such oldies as: (1) "We have the best health care system in the world," (2) "They have rationing and waiting lines in other countries," (3) "Why do so many people (especially Canadians) come here for their health care?" No one, however, seems to boast about the Saudi royal family coming here for care. It doesn't have the same ring. Then there is the ever-useful slur: (4) "They have socialized medicine," with the assumption that that must be bad, certainly un-American, and maybe even evil.

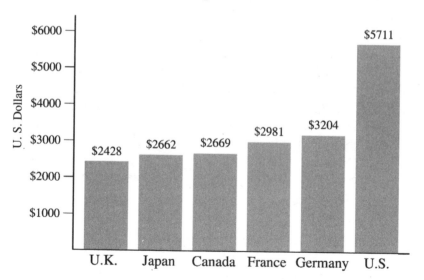

Per Capita Spending on Health Care – 2003

SOURCE: *The World Health Report, 2006.* World Health Organization.

Secondhand stories from friends or relatives in the other developed countries, notably Great Britain and Canada, tell mixed tales. Complaints about waiting lists for elective procedures, cancer treatment denied because someone was too old, controversial tabloid stories about emergency room disasters. There is an Idaho state senator who derides the Danish system for sending Danes to Mallorca in the winter for recovery and rehabilitation. I suspect it's cheaper, and more effective, to send people to recover in a warm climate than to keep them in a hospital in Denmark.

On the other hand, there are many stories that relate how far the systems in these other countries have gone to try to deliver the proper care. We hear of timely air evacuations in Canada or coordinated holistic home care for the elderly in Great Britain. Maybe older Brits aren't as likely to get a kidney transplant when they're in renal failure. But they're much more likely than their American counterparts to have regular home visits to assess their overall needs from a team including a doctor, a nurse, and a social worker.[5] And ask Brits or Canadians if they'd like to switch their health care system for ours, as I have, and the reply will be overwhelmingly negative (of course, there always are some exceptions).

Americans who have had personal contact with health care systems in other developed countries tell about a variety of experiences. Sometimes they have encountered bureaucratic red tape, other times access has been simple. Their experiences have usually been favorable. They have generally been impressed with the low cost of the care and how much more humane the care seemed in comparison with America. An Idaho physician related how when he was in Ireland and suffered a mini-stroke, he had easy access to care, but they didn't have the expensive clot-dissolving drug to administer to him. My niece, who had her third baby in Dublin at about the same time, feels that her maternity care in Ireland was vastly superior to the care she had received in Washington, D.C.

In an article entitled "So Lucky to Give Birth in England," which appeared in a *The New York Times* "Health and Fitness" section, an American woman who had a baby in London described her experience with the British system.[6] She subsequently had three more children in America. When friends ask her about her birthing experience in England, she tells them she "was lucky to be in London the first time around." Britain's National Health Service provided a daily home visit by a midwife for 10 days after the birth to check on mom and baby. She said that she "felt connected to a community, one that cared for its new babies and new mothers." With the birth of her last babies (twins) in New York City, she "was discharged within 48 hours and sent home to fend for [her]self."

David Burgess is a self-described American "right-winger" who works for *The Herald Tribune* in Paris. After receiving treatment for cancer of the esophagus in France, he wrote about his experience with the French health care system and related how he had been converted to the merits of "socialized medicine." He wound up paying $6.50 out of pocket for medical care that an American physician friend told him would have cost over a half million dollars in the United States. And Burgess praised the quality of care as excellent.

I've heard accounts from several Americans who were traveling abroad (specifically, stories from France, Spain, and Italy— as well as a personal one of my own from Switzerland). People relate how easy, and relatively inexpensive, it was to get care when they had an accident, usually a fracture. Some of them weren't even charged at all. And universally they note how they were treated with human kindness. That kind of caring happens in America too, but it seems to happen here with decreasing frequency. I hear in my mind the first question from the front desk, "Do you have insurance?"

Our Much-Maligned Neighbor to the North

CANADA, BECAUSE OF ITS PROXIMITY to the United States, has its own special spot in American mythology. They have long wait lists (not as much of a problem as it's presumed). It's socialized medicine (it isn't). Canadians are coming south "in droves"[7] for care (as opposed to the much larger number of Americans who go to Canada for cheaper medications or to have their babies). There are more CAT scanners in Peoria than in all of Canada (an exaggeration). Canadian ERs are falling apart under the demand (the same as in the United States, it turns out). Canadian doctors are abandoning Canada to come to the United States. (In fact, the trend is reversing. In 2005 the number of doctors going back to Canada actually exceeded the number coming south.)

No one has disputed the quality of care in Canada—it's agreed to be at least equal to the quality in the United States. And no one can legitimately complain about a lack of medical research in Canada. Canada produces at least as much research as does the United States—of course, in proportion to its population. Medical education in Canada is almost free, at least compared to the United States, and graduates don't have $100,000 loans to pay off when they leave medical school. When they go into practice, they don't have the same incentives as their American counterparts to make money in order to repay a huge debt.

But Canada's system has borne the brunt of negative advertising campaigns in the United States, campaigns that have been successful in coloring Americans' perceptions of the Canadian system. The American Medical Association spent several million dollars in the early '90s to discredit the Canadian system and create doubts in the mind of the American public about a government-managed system for universal coverage. And in 2000, in a somewhat less successful ad campaign that cost perhaps $60 million, the American pharmaceutical industry tried to discredit the Canadian system. A ubiquitous "bus from Canada" appeared in a plethora of TV spots and full-page newspaper ads across the United States. The goal was to derail efforts to make pharmaceutical benefits an integral part of Medicare.

The Canadian system has had its funding problems. It spends about half as much per capita on health care as we do; $2,669 per person compared to $5,711 per person in the United States. If one were to look at total health care spending as a percentage of GDP, Canada spends only 9.9 percent compared to 15.2 percent in the United States (2006 World Health Organization report using the latest 2003 figures). But despite problems with underfunding, the Canadians are able to cover every person with a fairly

comprehensive health care package, which does vary from
province to province as the system is not monolithic. And they
are fiercely proud of their universal coverage. I remember a
Toronto taxi driver (who had a foreign accent) holding up his
medicare card and waving it proudly when we asked him about
the Canadian health care system. "With this card I can get health
care anywhere I want," he proclaimed.

Frank and Ernest

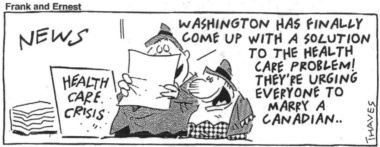

© 1995 Thaves / Reprinted with permission. Newspaper dist. by NEA, Inc.

Of course, there are Canadians who do complain. Complaining
is a way to get change in Canada, as it should be in any democracy. However, if we were to compare the degree of seriousness
of the complaints in Canada versus the United States, it would be
a "no contest." The U.S. "horror stories" would win hands down.
There is much we could learn from Canada[8] if so many of us
weren't so convinced that we had "the best health care system in
the world." The other developed countries have learned a lot from
each other, but we Americans automatically assume we have
nothing to learn from the experience of others.

Our Ranking in the World

WHEN WE USE OBJECTIVE CRITERIA to compare our
system to those of the other developed countries, we rank far
from "best"—except in the area of spending, where we're way
ahead of anyone else. As related in Chapter 1, the 2000 World
Health Organization study that rated health systems of the world
gave the United States 37th ranking in overall health system performance, a long way from number one. One can argue about the
criteria that were used, but there's no doubt that in the category

of "fairness," which played a heavy role in the rankings, we do very poorly. In fact, in the specific category of "fairness," we tied for 54th place with Fiji.

How about health outcomes? When we compare the United States to other countries, using the WHO standards in the so-called "Health Care Olympics," the final U.S. standings in the 2005 WHO report are nothing short of damning: life expectancy, 27th; maternal mortality, 29th; infant mortality, 35th; mortality before the age of 5, 36th; percentage of the population over age 60, 40th. Our immunization rates for children are even worse! In fact, Cuba, Croatia, and Kazakhstan have better immunization rates for measles in children under the age of 2 than the country that boasts "The greatest health care system in the world." The *only* place where the United States of America ranks number one is in the total amount of money spent per capita and the percentage of Gross Domestic Product spent on health care! The fact that we're by far number one in health care spending should raise some doubts about the value we Americans get for the amount of money we spend on health care. In all fairness, however, our poor showing for the standard health outcome measures is likely as much a result of America's wide social and economic disparities as our dysfunctional health care system. But given these wide disparities, the argument for universal coverage is even stronger.

We need to quit putting our collective heads in the sand as we blithely dismiss ideas from other nations, even the developing world. When I worked to help develop a primary health care system in Swaziland in 1989, we had an information system that gave us better data than I get in the United States today. Swaziland even had more options for birth control then because Depo-Provera was not yet being used in America. Yet because we assume we are "the best"—and have been encouraged to keep believing that assumption by the medical-industrial complex—we fail to look outside the United States for ideas. We need to acknowledge that our health care financing system is unfair, unjust, fragmented, expensive, wasteful, and broken. And that it behooves us to look north—and even south, west, and east—to learn how to improve our system so that it can be affordable and accessible to every person in America.

Summary of Key Points

- Americans are highly misinformed about the health care situation in other countries.

- America far exceeds the amount of money spent (per capita) on health care compared to all the other developed nations of the world; yet, as a population, our outcomes are worse.

- All the other industrialized countries have universal coverage.

- America is the only developed country where getting sick or injured can, and all too frequently does, lead to bankruptcy.

PART TWO

Toward Finding a Solution

"We need to unite, get together, and demand universal coverage."

— A 62-year-old patient at my health center

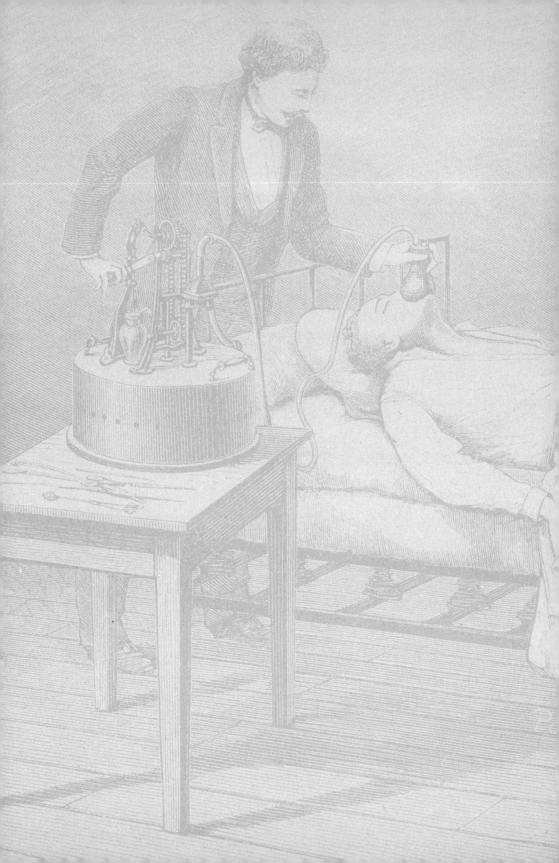

Chapter 11

The Price of Health:
How Much Should We Americans
Be Spending on Health Care?

My wife's "Aunt" Selma relates how her long-deceased husband, a pediatrician, used to help indigent patients back in the 1940s, when an office visit was $3. "He'd just take care of them and not worry about the payment. And he'd take care of patients at the free clinic and accept barter. That's the way it was."

WE'VE COME A LONG WAY since the Good Old Days, since the days when few people had (or needed to have) health insurance. Health care was a cottage industry. Most physicians were individual professionals practicing medicine as a labor of love and service. Medicine wasn't a bad living, but physicians—or for that matter, hospital administrators, many of whom were Catholic nuns—were not earning a fortune. Group practices, the few that existed, were reviled by the American Medical Association (AMA) as creeping socialism. General practitioners, like the fabled Marcus Welby, were icons in their communities. There were no expensive medicines or procedures. Nurses did nursing. Hospitals were mostly supported and run by communities or religious groups, not corporations. No one shunned "charity" care. It was a responsibility felt by almost every community and every physician.

In the early '40s, the charge for a physician's home delivery in rural Idaho was $40. Even in 1975, when I started an 8-year stint as a private solo-practice family doctor in Nampa, Idaho, my charge for the regular office visit was $9. For a brief visit, it was $6.

In 1971, when I first became interested in health policy issues, the United States spent $70 billion a year on health care. That amount was then considered excessive, and Nixon's administration came up with the idea of promoting health maintenance organizations (HMOs), styled after the Kaiser plan, to control Medicare and Medicaid spending. In 2006 annual health expenditures will exceed $2 trillion—nearly a 30-fold increase from 1971 and more than a 30 percent increase from 2001 (when the first edition of this book was printed).

When I first opened my private practice in 1975, I decided (an economic gamble) to go without health insurance for my family and myself. We were young and healthy. And, at least in those days, physicians' fees for a doctor and his family were written off as medical courtesy. Economically, the gamble paid off. During the 5 years we were uninsured, I would have paid about $5,000 for health insurance. And in those years we only incurred one expense of note. My 8-year-old son, attempting to simultaneously daydream and ride no-hands on his bike, fell and broke his arm. The fracture had to be set under general anesthesia. The hospital bill, including the operating room charge, came to about $300. The physicians, as was customary in those days, extended medical courtesy. Today, the operating room charges alone would be a few thousand dollars.

Although there is a small movement today by a handful of physicians and others (such as nurse practitioners) to set back the clock by practicing cut-rate cash-only ambulatory medicine, health care is no longer a cottage industry. The Good Old Days are long gone.

Of course, the Good Old Days weren't necessarily that good for everybody. For example, hospital workers were usually paid a minimum wage—in 1962, around $1 an hour. For them, that meant living in or near poverty. Medical interns and residents were paid $250 a month for a 120-hour workweek, a practice that persisted until they banded together in the mid-'60s to demand a living wage. When some interns applied for welfare, and qualified, the hospitals gave in. Then there were the pre-Medicare days, when a great number of seniors stayed in poverty because of medical bills or simply went without medical care.

Medicare, after Social Security, became perhaps the most important solution to poverty for seniors. Medicare permitted retirees to live with dignity. Both Medicare and Medicaid made it possible for low-income elderly people and the poor to avoid becoming "health care beggars." Simultaneously, these programs helped support the hospitals and physicians who took care of them. Moreover, these two government programs led to social change. They mandated changes in civil rights like the desegregation of hospital wards. Prior to Medicare, in the early 1960s, the medical wards at the Johns Hopkins Hospital, where I trained, were segregated into separate floors for blacks and whites.

The "Good Old Days" Are Over

HEALTH CARE IN THE UNITED STATES has long ceased to be a cottage industry. The change has been especially rapid over the past two decades. With rapidly rising costs and the squeezing of providers by managed care, financing health care for the uninsured has become progressively more problematic. Charity care, despite the barely measurable effect of "free clinics," has nearly vanished from the health care scene. To a great extent, so has the notion of "charity." Even for the insured, it can be a hard world. We saw an insured woman in her twenties with abdominal pain whom we referred to a surgeon for possible appendicitis. When she got to the surgeon's front desk, she was told she didn't have the proper referral forms required by her insurance company. She spent the next 2 hours crying in pain in her car in the parking lot. Luckily, she got better. It probably wasn't appendicitis.

The old practice of cost-shifting that allowed excess receipts from insured patients to cover the costs of the uninsured or indigent has largely disappeared. The excess receipts virtually evaporated or were pared down by: (1) "Diagnosis Related Groups" (DRGs), where hospitals were paid by diagnosis, not cost; and (2) penny-pinching HMO contracts foisted on hospitals under the threat of losing their market share. However, with the recent collapse of managed care, the HMOs have lost much of their clout with the hospitals. It remains to be seen what will happen with charity care, but some hospitals, including our local hospital in

Nampa, Idaho, have been more willing to write off some charges up front. Perhaps they realized they would be unable to collect anyway.

Specialists, meanwhile, have become less willing to write off the cost of consultations and procedures. Their business managers tell them they can't do it, and their front desks turn the uninsured patients away if they can't plunk down a large amount of cash up front. It has become increasingly difficult for cash-poor uninsured people to get specialist care. More recently, it has also become harder for cash-poor insured people to get the care they need because of the ever-increasing deductibles and co-pays. And as employers go in the direction of "defined contributions" (a euphemism for cost-shifting) by providing only high-deductible plans with health savings accounts, out-of-pocket health expenditures will only increase for employees.[1] The result will be that even middle-class insured Americans will find themselves in a more difficult bind.

Costs Are Going Up, Up, Up

A LARGE PART OF our current problem stems from the increasing cost of health care. As mentioned above, U.S. spending on health care went from about $70 billion in 1971 to over $2 trillion in 2006. At the time this book was first published, the Centers for Medicare & Medicaid Services (CMS) released a report that predicted health care spending would double between 2002 and 2011 to a total of $2.8 trillion.[2] This would represent a per capita spending of more than $9,200 and consume 17 percent of our GDP. At our current pace, we may reach those numbers by 2009.

Premiums for private health insurance have risen even faster and continue to exceed the average annual increase in national health care spending. A report released in January 2006 by the Office of the Actuary for the CMS shows that total health care spending "cooled" somewhat to 7.9 percent but that premiums for private health insurance rose by 8.6 percent. This is actually the first time in several years that increases have fallen below double digits, but it still outpaces the growth of our economy by two to three times!

Some major factors responsible for the soaring costs of health care include an aging population, technological advances, increasing administrative costs, wasteful duplication of services, and an inflated pricing system. High consumer expectations, fueled by corporate advertising, media hype, and the Internet, also have contributed to the rising costs of health care, as has the cost of so-called "defensive medicine." But undoubtedly the most significant reason for skyrocketing costs has been new technology. A double-edged sword. While usually expensive, new technological advances have been both wonderful and incredible in terms of how they have affected our lives and our health. Here are but a few examples of the positive effects of new technology:

- Joint replacements now allow older people to lead more fulfilling, less painful, and more active lives in their senior years.

- Bleeding or perforated ulcers, and their accompanying mortality, are now rare because of new medicines that suppress gastric acid secretion.

- Many operations are now much simpler, with less pain and much quicker recovery times, thanks to laparoscopic surgery and other microsurgical techniques.

- Intensive care for newborns saves tiny premature babies—babies who only 25 years ago were left to die because they were considered too small to survive.

- Many heart attacks are now prevented by the placement of stents in narrowed coronary arteries.

- Many more people with mental illness can now be treated outside hospitals because of new, more effective antipsychotic and antidepressant medications.

Many of these advances, like the drugs that inhibit gastric acid secretion and have reduced the need for ulcer surgery, very likely have made health care *less* expensive. Blood chemistry panels have become incredibly *in*expensive—pennies a test—

because of new techniques. But by vastly expanding the possibilities, new technologies have made medical care more expensive. In many cases, the technological advances (such as joint replacements) have made possible therapies that were unavailable in the past. A worn-out hip? In the old days, treatment might have been limited to a shot of cortisone and a walker. Do we need to return to those days because we can no longer afford to pay for hip replacements? Or should we consider saving $3,000 by substituting a less-expensive artificial hip joint that only carries a 5-year warranty?

Despite their cost, many of the new technologies offer some theoretical long-term savings. Joint replacements are effective for keeping the elderly out of nursing homes. The new "statin" drugs, though expensive themselves, will likely prevent millions of heart attacks and strokes, all of which are expensive to treat. However, the cost-benefit analyses for many of these new modalities usually don't show them to be cost saving in the "big picture." Sometimes the large number of interventions necessary to avoid a smaller number of catastrophes doesn't always balance out financially. For example, the universal administration of flu vaccine in the workplace has been shown to not be cost-effective. A failing of these cost/benefit studies, however, is that they usually do not factor in quality-of-life considerations. What is a week of good health without the flu worth?

A February 2002 study from the National Bureau of Economic Research by Yale economist William D. Nordhaus, however, suggested "the social productivity of health care spending might be many times that of other spending."[3] Maybe 17 percent of the GDP isn't too much. Nordhaus questioned the current feeling that our health care system is "stupendously wasteful" compared to other economic activities—at least when it comes to the overall benefits accrued to society. The finding is inherent in the nature of health care (it doesn't take an economist to appreciate the old adage that "if you don't have your health, you don't have anything"), but it doesn't excuse the internal wastefulness, injustice, and craziness of our current system.

Ethics—and Profits vs. Patients

BEYOND THE ISSUE OF pure cost, the new technologies have raised a host of ethical concerns. Cost is certainly a societal issue when we perform microsurgeries on babies' hearts inside the mother's uterus—at a cost of a half million dollars. Or when we save babies that weigh less than 2 pounds—at a cost of a few hundred thousand dollars. These same tiny babies have a high incidence of neurological damage later and require more resources. What about spending close to a million dollars (as the state of California is doing) for a heart transplant for a state prison inmate?

And how about our spending at the end of life? Should we be spending large sums of money in often-futile efforts to prolong life for the terminally ill elderly? End-of-life costs for medical care in America are considerable but often overstated. The actual estimate reflecting this cost is that 30 percent of Medicare spending goes to the beneficiaries of that program in their last year of life.

Where do we draw a line? Is that process called setting priorities—or rationing? When we didn't have the advanced technology, we did what we could as caregivers to alleviate pain and suffering. But now we must deal with the ethical issues involved with expensive measures such as bone marrow transplants, organ transplants, and other costly treatments for illnesses that cost hundreds of thousands of dollars or more. Some of the treatments have been shown to have questionable value, such as bone marrow transplants for breast cancer or extremely expensive antibiotics (a million dollars' worth) to treat Lyme disease.

The high-ticket items are the ones we usually hear debated. But, as any insurance actuary will tell you, these financial disasters are relatively rare. Including them in an insurance plan does not really add much to the cost of premiums—if there's a very large "risk pool." In contrast, the way clinicians practice everyday medicine involves hundreds of millions of patient encounters. And we clinicians are incredibly wasteful in our practice of everyday health care. A large part of the huge expense we incur is in excessive pricing. But much too large a part is in our failure to practice scientifically based medicine. Why should a young person with a first-time urinary tract infection be prescribed Cipro, which costs $100, when a $10 drug works just as well? Is it necessary that an echocardiogram (at $1,200) be done for a healthy older person getting a cardiac evaluation? How often, and with what indications, should colonoscopy (at $2,000) be done? What about liver biopsies (at $3,000) for hepatitis C? Does every neck injury require an X-ray and/or a CAT scan? How many skin lesions (at $200 a whack) does the dermatologist really need to remove?

The conscientious (for some the word would be "zealous") specialist wants to be "complete." And she/he has a "stable" of costly procedures that (1) bring in good income and (2) make the patients feel they have been treated well. It's a three-part game of physician zeal (and, sometimes, greed), high patient expectations, and overpriced procedures/medications.

The "good part" of managed care was supposed to be about controlling these factors. But managed care got diverted into putting cost factors and profits first—despite the lip service to caring about people. As for practicing scientifically based medicine with a consideration for cost-effectiveness, America's health care is not yet there. Interestingly enough, some of the most practical work in using a scientific approach to diagnostic testing has come from Canada. The Canadians have developed objective guidelines, for example, to decide when and if X-rays are necessary for two common situations: ankle and neck injuries.

Another sticky wicket, which has yet to receive much press, is in the area of genetic testing. Science is now able to map the entire human genome. Armed with this information, breaking the secrets of the human genetic code is within our grasp. We already understand the genetic information of many cancers and inherited diseases, but what we know today is a mere trifle compared to what we will be able to do in the not too distant future. There will come a time, which most of us will live to see, when we will collect a small sample of blood or tissue from a newborn and be able to predict with great accuracy that child's propensity for diabetes, high blood pressure, Alzheimer's disease, cancer, etc. What an incredible tool at our disposal! Armed with that information, we can begin to intervene from day one to minimize, or prevent altogether, all kinds of human maladies to which we are genetically prone.

One example is the BRCA 1 and BRCA 2 tumor suppressor genes identified with breast cancer. More than 100 mutations of these genes have already been described, and they can be passed to both male and female children. We know that if a woman carries a mutation for either one of these genes and has a family history of breast or ovarian cancer; by the age of 50 she will have at least a 50 percent chance of developing breast cancer or a 30 percent chance of developing ovarian cancer. Although treatment options are controversial, we can reduce the likelihood of a young woman developing these cancers with surgical intervention. Herein lies the rub.

First off, many private insurance carriers do not pay for genetic screening, but even more important, if they find out that a patient carries a gene of a potentially catastrophic disease, they will do everything in their power to keep from insuring the individual. And if the patient is covered, they will look for every opportunity to drop the person like a hot potato!

I have a colleague whose wife developed breast cancer in her late forties. Her oncologist suggested that her daughter, who was in her mid-twenties at the time, be tested for a BRCA mutation. She tested positive and made the heart-wrenching decision to undergo surgery to remove both her breasts. This otherwise perfectly healthy young woman with a college degree and a professional career now is uninsurable for the rest of her life. No private insurance carrier will even give her the time of day.

Now, I can't say that I blame them. After all, if you are going to make a profit in the insurance industry, you have to minimize your exposure to high-risk patients. But that's the problem—profit.

If there is only one concept that the reader takes away after returning this book to the shelf, it is simply this: A profit-based, market-driven system and equitable, quality health care cannot be, and never will be, compatible. Not now, not ever!

But the story of this young woman is only the beginning. As our ability to predict disease using genetic (as well as other markers) improves, we have the opportunity to intervene and enhance the health of individuals as well as society. But that information is now, and will be, used against us all in a market-driven system. Traditionally, insurance carriers have used population-based actuarial tables to calculate risk. They can use any number of population groups when setting premiums—from an entire state all the way down to a small business of 15 employees. But as our ability to predict disease in individuals improves, the market will be forced to set individual risk and ratings (even at birth). Many will be born uninsurable!

The only way for an insurance company to continue to make a profit in this setting is to glean the genetically perfect (if there is such a thing), make higher-risk patients pay more for their genes, or be subsidized with taxpayer money. It's no wonder that the current policy in Washington, driven by a huge deep-pocket lobby of for-profit insurance carriers, is pushing for "personal responsibility." In so doing, they can increase their profit margins by offering high-deductible plans (cost-shifting), encouraging legislators to provide insurance through tax vouchers (which are nothing more than government subsidies), and shoving high-risk patients over to government programs.

Private for-profit insurance companies are not in the business of providing quality, innovative delivery of health care. They are in the business of making money—period!

American researchers, such as the Agency for Healthcare Research and Quality (AHRQ)[4] and the U.S. Preventive Services Task Force, are also busy developing guidelines. The latter entity applies a scientific approach to the analysis of preventive measures. Their recommendations are often critical of a host of costly, and even invasive, procedures advocated by some other groups. America's specialty groups, such as the surgeons, the gastroenterologists, and the gynecologists, tend to be more aggressive in their advice. Well-meaning as these specialists are, their viewpoint (often from a scope that gets threaded into a small orifice) might be called "narrow"—literally and figuratively.

How do we as a society decide what we will pay for? And how much are we willing to pay for those services?

Health policy expert Jonathan Weiner asserts that what America needs is "an accountable, transparent mechanism that makes use of scientific evidence, ethics, and consumer values to collectively decide what we can and cannot afford to cover as a basic insurance package."[5] For so-called "marginal" services, he adds, people could have optional coverage or pay out of pocket. He summarizes, "No industrialized nation spends more than America on medical care, excludes more of its citizens from coverage, and is less rational in the way it sets its spending priorities."

In the United States, these financial choices have often been dictated more by politics and profits—or even happenstance—than by need. Why does Medicare automatically cover people with kidney dialysis? There must be hundreds of other conditions that deserve equal treatment. What about "Jerry's kids"? There is a host of other disorders that merit hoopla equal to that lavished upon muscular dystrophy. Yet periodically we are beseeched at the checkout stands of supermarkets and at street corners by well-meaning people collecting money for this specific, and relatively uncommon, ailment. Not to mention the telethons. American-style health care financing—and prioritizing.

"Expecting the World"

PEOPLE IN THE UNITED STATES, at least if they have insurance, have come to "expect the world" from health care. How can you put a price on a child's life, especially if it's *your* child? How much is it worth to save a spouse who just had a heart attack? I no longer hear the kind of request I used to hear fairly frequently a decade or two ago, the request to "do everything possible—the cost doesn't matter"—to save 88-year-old grandpa. There has been a transformation in American society in our attitude towards death and dying, at least for the aged. I almost never see a living will now where an elderly person asks for extraordinary measures to preserve life. But it's totally different for younger folks.

People's expectations have been fueled and sustained by a corporate culture that has used "the market" to help create a society that "expects the world" from medical care. The sky's the limit from the new technologies—in terms of both an array of wonderful possibilities and (unfortunately) cost. Unlimited dreams, and unlimited profits, have helped create an American ethic, consistent with the free-enterprise spirit, that downplays the role of cost. Modern-day "snake oil merchants" are not only hawking an array of useful and not-always-so-useful products. They have also created a whole framework of myths and misinformation to assure their continued profits. And they have had huge influence over the media, which benefit financially from lavish spending on advertising.

This same corporate world has had a huge influence, through politics and lobbyists, on what direction American health care has taken. For the pharmaceutical industry, their campaign contributions and lobbying efforts have been rewarded with such perks as extended times for patents (Prilosec, for example) and generous tax write-offs. The doctors (at least specialists) have managed to keep their fees high. And the insurance industry has (so far) been able to raise its premiums and exclude high-risk clients with little opposition.

As explained above, there was a brief period in the mid-1990s—in the heyday of the "managed-care revolution"—when the increase in health care costs seemed to flatten out. But at the end of the last decade, the HMO "bad guys" retreated. However, they could stage a comeback, as once again America is experiencing double-digit inflation in the cost of health care.

Did Americans really get what they wished for, as Princeton health economist Uwe Reinhardt has inferred?[6] Many Americans who bought into the expectation of health care without limits got tired of being restrained and abused by managed care. They helped make the HMOs back away from limiting care. Perhaps the HMOs, playing a competitive game that artificially lowered health care spending, realized that they could no longer profitably play the same game. They have been leaving Medicare managed care because the profits weren't there. Meanwhile, in all the maneuvering, they have not made patient interests a high priority. Leaving patients high and dry doesn't seem to matter, as the HMOs and insurance companies, like Aetna, seem to be starting to abandon the sinking ship of managed care, especially with regard to Medicare.

The Future, Technology, and Costs

THE HEALTH CARE INDUSTRY has largely played to the individual American's pursuit of personal happiness (with health, and all the trimmings). There has been little sense of responsibility to the community. In the Good Old Days, the center of most Americans' health care world was their general practitioner and their community hospital. Today, the focus has shifted to powerful insurance companies, mega-clinics, and giant HMOs, all of which have become increasingly for-profit. It's amazing how modern-day corporate health care has changed even the way Americans use language to frame the issues. It used to be that we had free choice of physician. Now we are told we need more choice of plan. And physicians didn't use to be "providers." It blows my mind to think that so many of us physicians have come to accept our being referred to as "providers" without throwing open our exam-room doors and shouting, "I'm mad as hell, and I'm not going to take this anymore!"

The Good Old Days were when health care did not comprise one-seventh of the whole U.S. economy. Those days were before corporate America woke up and noticed that there was money to be made and fat to be trimmed in a sector of the economy that was huge and naïve to market forces. Health care had, and still has, the potential for a huge profit margin, as the pharmaceutical companies, the medical equipment manufacturers, and certain subspecialist physicians have learned.

There are still major market forces poised to "make a killing" in health care. The possibilities for profit coming from new technologies are immense. There is probably no other sector of the American economy that offers so much potential for profit. The American public has been primed for "endless health." It has become accustomed to having someone else pay for its health care. And it has been immunized against the forces of constraint, such as regulators and health care reformers, through the lobbying efforts and advertising campaigns of the medical-industrial establishment.

Will the ever-increasing spiral of health care costs ever end? At what point should it be slowed down or capped? What percentage of our GDP should be consumed by health care? Is 30 percent, as some have predicted, too much?

An immediate danger of rising costs is the threat they present to the viability of Medicare and Medicaid. With a worsening economy, state and federal budget-watchers will have an excuse to gut these programs.

Some of our cost factors are clearly wasteful, illogical, and exploitative. Pricing is crazy. There is an excess of administrative burden and waste. Our preoccupation with individual health and curative medicine has led us down the path of expensive cures when we should be investing much more in prevention, both on an individual and a societal basis. The path of prevention and community-centered health can be a force for lower costs, greater fairness, and affordability. And, if we were to embrace universal coverage, we would reap further savings by largely eliminating delayed or omitted care, which lead to more serious and expensive interventions.

We can do nothing about the aging of our population, the greater number of elderly who will need health services. However, if our public health and preventive programs were effective, we could see people aging with fewer disabilities from chronic disease. There would be less heart disease, emphysema, diabetes, obesity, and joint disease secondary to obesity, etc. People wouldn't require as much expensive remedial care, like cardiac stents, bypass surgery, or joint replacements.

Prevention, specifically community-oriented prevention, is the path to choose. But prevention will have to compete for dollars with new technologies. And right now, the medical-industrial complex is putting its money on new technologies, not prevention. A paradigm shift toward prevention is in order (see Chapter 17).

David Callahan, in his book *False Hopes: Why America's Quest for Perfect Health Is a Recipe for Failure,*[7] labels the new technologies and the medical paradigm of conquering disease and death as "false hopes." He supports the public health approach as well as the strengthening of our inner selves. I agree—and partially disagree.

Having experienced medicine in the age prior to our current wave of new technologies, I can say that I have seen some near-miracles in what some (but not all) of these advances have meant to people's lives. The 80-year-old woman who, facing invalidism in her final years, can suddenly play golf again with her new hip joint. Or the woman who avoided major surgery by having a cancerous polyp removed from her colon via colonoscopy. The hundreds of my patients who can live normal lives again because new, and more effective, antidepressants are available.

The new technologies hold great promise for the future, for future cures, and for prevention. If we could put at least as much money into developing new public health and preventive technologies, we would be better serving the interests of America. So I would agree with David Callahan that we should divert a good part of our investment from research on the expensive, limited-use technology to the kind of technologies that can benefit whole communities. It's common sense, not socialism.

What about those Americans who have either (1) relatively rare diseases or (2) an ailment or injury that is very expensive to treat? Should they be denied the kind of advances that come with potential new technologies, like gene therapy? Should this new kind of technology be limited to the rich, who can pay for it with their own money?

Then there are the unfortunate people who have a combination of (1) and (2), a rare disease that is very expensive to treat. Such was the case of 19-year-old Brandy Stroeder (she has since died), an Oregon woman with cystic fibrosis who needed a heart/lung/liver transplant. The Oregon Health Plan, which covered her insurance, would not pay for the surgery she needed because "health plan officials argue[d] that the procedure is experimental and that funding must be reserved for primary and preventative services."[8] Oregon led the nation in trying to come up with a form of "rationing" of health care. For Oregon Medicaid patients, a list of diagnoses and treatments was drawn up with each item prioritized in order. Depending on available budget resources, a line is drawn on that list. The Oregon Health Plan reimburses items above that line. Below the line, the Plan won't cover it. Yes, it's rationing. And it was a methodology developed with careful and full community input. The reality is that, given limited public funds and unlimited technological advances, "rationing" of some sort is necessary—even in America, where "we don't want rationing." How should we Americans deal with the issue? What would have been the right decision for Brandy Stroeder?

The Answer Needs to Come From the People

I DON'T HAVE THE answer. But I feel the answer should come from the American people as a community. We should have the right as a community to decide where we put our pooled resources. Assuming we are well informed, and that is a large assumption, we should have input in deciding what projects should be researched by our National Institutes of Health, for example. If we decide, as a community, that we want to spend millions of dollars to seek a cure for a disease that only one of us has, because that's the kind of inclusiveness we feel as a community, then so be it. Or if we feel, as a nation, that we need to give more attention to researching alternative medicine, then we should be able to do that. If we decide, as a community, that we want to spend 30 percent of our GDP on health care (and, hopefully, public health and prevention get included), then that's okay. We'll have to spend less on other things. An article in the Business section of *The New York Times*[9] raised the issue of whether health care should become the driver of the American economy. Goodbye, General Motors and Exxon Mobil.

A major potential problem in expanding health care to such a huge percentage of our economy is the concern about getting value for our investment. If the history of health care costs to date is any measure of our success, we've failed. We've gotten poor value for our bucks. Unless we tie increased investment in our health care sector with a major paradigm shift to public health and prevention—and better outcomes—we'll be throwing away our money.

The problem with the community process for setting priorities is the likelihood of its being tainted by the vested health care interests and their myths. They have consistently used their influence, media campaigns, lobbyists, or campaign contributions to get the results they want, the results that will protect and enhance their financial interests. Given today's political reality, it may take some other very basic measures, such as campaign finance reform, to allow the community process to work. It will not be an easy task (see the following chapter) for Americans to win meaningful health care reform and affordable health care with such a powerful array of corporate interests blocking the way.

Meanwhile, if we are to prioritize some expensive new technologies, how about an artificial heart for the insurance industry? Maybe then, they'd care about us.

Summary of Key Points

- The cost of America's health care continues to escalate at a rate considerably above the rate of inflation.

- New technologies are the major factor driving the higher costs even as they make some interventions more affordable.

- We get poor value in America for the money we spend on health care.

- With our escalating costs, we need to invest a much greater proportion of our health care dollars in prevention and public health.

- As a nation, we need to make our expectations more consistent with how much we are willing to spend on health care versus other expenditures.

- Health care has the potential to become "the driver" of our economy.

Don Quixote vs. the Establishment: Can the Medical-Industrial Complex Be Toppled?

On the cover of the December 9, 2001, Chicago Tribune Magazine is a full-page color photo of a thoughtful-appearing Quentin Young, MD. Large letters across the picture read, "Doc Quixote." The subscript: "For 50 years, Quentin Young has pushed for health care for all. Will he ever realize his dream?"

"The [health care] system is controlled by a small handful of powerful people, economic forces, whose profit-making takes precedence over the national, and indeed, the world cause of good health."[1]
—Rep. John Conyers (D-MI)

MOVED BY A DESIRE to improve access to health care in America, in 1990 I decided to run for the Idaho State Legislature. As a result, some of my colleagues compared me to Don Quixote tilting at windmills. Years later, I reflected upon those windmills as I rode past a huge complex of hospitals near downtown Denver. I gazed with awe at the large illuminated signs on the sides of the towering buildings. These guys are big, rich, and powerful. And they have powerful friends and allies, like the insurance companies, the pharmaceutical industry, and organized medicine. They can drop a few million dollars to try to kill a ballot initiative in California or Massachusetts—or a referendum in Portland, Maine. Against such odds, how much chance did I have to shake up the "medical-industrial complex"? The forces to oppose change control one-seventh of our economy. And there I was, gazing up at these huge monoliths of power. Don Quixote. A community health center physician serving mostly low-wage uninsured patients who pay a $10 nominal fee for a visit. Fortunately, Quentin Young, and others like him, are on our side.

Health care in America has evolved into an incredibly complex entity. Our system is so fragmented and complicated that it's almost impossible to comprehend. It's easy to plant doubt ("There must be a better way") in the public mind, doubt that will make people wary of change. It's also easy, when you have lots of money, to create and perpetuate myths that protect the status quo. In the face of such powerful opposition, what can we Don Quixotes do to fix our fragmented, costly, and inequitable system, a system that excludes one-seventh of our population from adequate access to care? Can we do something to improve our dismal near-to-last ranking among the developed countries for almost every health indicator?

"The Evil Empire": How Bad Is It?

THE U.S. DEPARTMENT OF HEALTH AND HUMAN SERVICES has an initiative, "Zero Disparities," linked to *Healthy People 2010*, to eliminate all health care disparities. It's extremely unlikely to happen unless America has universal coverage. To quote Rep. Donna Christian-Christensen (D-VI), "There can be no elimination of disparities if everyone . . . does not have insurance coverage."[2] And America will never have meaningful or affordable universal coverage as long as the powerful vested interests hold sway over what happens to health care in America. The uninsured and the folks on the low end of the disparity gulf have probably less than one-tenth of 1 percent of the lobbying resources available to the "Gang of Four" (pharmaceutical industry, insurance industry, hospitals, and organized medicine) that comprises "the Evil Empire" of health care. The combined campaign contributions of health care's Gang of Four are unrivaled.

Incidentally, when I use the term "Evil Empire," I am by no means implying that the people associated with these groups are bad. The overwhelming majority of the people working for the Gang of Four are sincere, well-meaning, good people. They're just clueless. They're caught up in the complexity of the system and unaware of the disastrous effects their business dealings are having upon many millions of Americans. They have little appreciation that their quest for "market share" and healthy bottom lines is making "health care beggars" out of millions of Americans and robbing them of their dignity.

What's really wrong is the value system that we have come to accept as a society. It's a value system that has helped create— and sustain—"the Evil Empire." It might be called the "Enron" paradigm. Push the legal envelope in the name of free enterprise. If you occasionally cross to the wrong side of the legal system, you pay your fines and continue on. Unless you're an Enron and go bankrupt, of course. It doesn't matter how many people are hurt in the process. If millions must go without heat or air conditioning because energy prices soar, and a few older folks die in the process, well, that's "the market." And the government will find some temporary solution to deal with the people who are most vulnerable, right?

Health care poses a similar situation. The parallel is uncanny. Millions go without health care because they can't afford it. People die because they delay care. And an ethic sanitizes the process by asserting, "That's just the effect of 'the market.'" Profits before patients because we believe in free enterprise, and, in the long run, "the market" will solve the problem. "Personal responsibility" for the consumer, but the primacy of self-interest for the Gang of Four. Lip service to universal coverage (it sounds altruistic), but keep the status quo so our bottom line isn't threatened. That's hypocrisy.

But it's worse. "The Evil Empire" has its plotters and their henchmen. They're not quite the same as the out-and-out crooks who use electronic chicanery to collect on services that were never delivered to patients. But it's sort of like "soft" porn. Overbilling for home health services. Systematic up-coding of diagnoses so third-party payers will pay more for services. Rationalizing expensive procedures or surgeries for patients who don't really need them. Using "creative accounting" to write off marketing expenses as health education. Lobbying legislators to push agendas that are shady. Writing legislation for them that protects practices that are marginal but profitable. The list goes on. The captains of industry begin to look more and more like pirates. And our society either (1) accepts all this highway robbery as "part of business as usual" or (2) is totally clueless. Unfortunately, both apply.

We modern-day Don Quixotes, like Quentin Young, have realized that the system is broken and corrupt. And what we're basically fighting, like Cervantes' Don Quixote, is a whole culture. We're committed to a similar quest, righting a wrong that too few around us perceive to be wrong. Our information system today is a little more sophisticated than the seventeenth-century novel. It's easier to get our word out. But it's also easier for the Gang of Four to buy a few million dollars of media time to cloud the issue. Or to make sure that symposia and proposals that deal with getting to universal coverage include poison pills—for example, "must be pluralistic"—that protect the status quo.

Toppling the Windmills

PERPETUATING THE CURRENT COMPLEX SYSTEM clearly fits the financial interests of the Gang of Four, or so they think. It allows them the potential to find opportunities for profit by manipulating the system. There are exceptions, some industry players who haven't totally forgotten about the needs of patients. But, generally speaking, as America's health care system has evolved, patient interests have largely been secondary to financial and business interests.

If we were to have comprehensive reform that had universal coverage with "one risk pool" and affordable, comprehensive care, the Gang of Four could be adversely affected financially. For starters, the pharmaceutical companies would be subject to group purchasing. Their worst nightmare, even beyond pharmaceutical benefits becoming an integral part of Medicare, would be to have all Americans covered with one risk pool. Either way, group purchasing power could cut their profits in half, or there could be price controls for drugs. As for the insurance companies, their cut of the health care pie, which now provides them with hefty commissions and profits, would be almost eliminated. They would be relegated to administrative duties, much as they do with Medicare today.

For physicians, medical subspecialists could see their incomes drop. There would be pressure to have more realistic pricing for their services. The historical over-reimbursement for medical and surgical procedures would change. As for the hospitals, the for-profits would need to worry about reduced bottom lines or convert to not-for-profit status. All hospitals, however, should welcome change that would help cover the costs of the uninsured patients they currently care for anyway.

I remember when a small group of people (including myself) from an organization that was then called the Idaho Citizens' Network put together a single-payer universal coverage health care reform bill for Idaho in 1991. We even managed to get an Idaho state senator to sponsor it and introduce the plan, called "IdaHealth," as legislation. A few people still kid me about how the bill failed in the Senate by a vote of 42–0. But when it came out, it caused a mild panic among the leaders of the health establishment. Fax machines (this was in the days before e-mail) fairly burned up in the establishment's quest to get the word out to defeat the plan.

In my idealistic and naïve hopes, as a (then) member of the Board of Trustees of the Idaho Medical Association, I tried to convince my fellow trustees (at least) not to oppose the legislation. Fat chance. It wasn't particularly difficult to get the Medical Association to endorse universal coverage as a concept (words are easy and cheap), but an actual bill was too much of a threat. The old war cry of "socialized medicine" rang out, and some physician friends referred to me as "their favorite communist."

What will it take to knock down the windmills? Actually, unless we have some cataclysmic event (and September 11 comes close), I don't think we Don Quixotes have much of a chance to defeat the forces of the Gang of Four—at least not by any frontal attack. The arguments for health care as a right, social justice, or compassion will continue to be countered by well-meaning (though sometimes greedy) people who will argue for "personal responsibility," market solutions, and for-profit schemes disguised as "more choice." The events of September 11 and the subsequent fear (and reality) of bioterrorism have created some heightened sense of community in America. The tragedy also may have mitigated the tendency for many Americans to espouse the ideals of "everyone for himself"—or, in the health care rhetoric, "personal responsibility." But idealism is probably not the "silver bullet" for meaningful reform. Economics most likely is.

Appealing to Self-Interest— Does It Have a Chance?

APPEALING TO THE CONSCIENCES of the Gang of Four will probably do little to eliminate the windmills, though it's certainly important to have a strong philosophical basis to support the reasons for health care reform. And it's key that we have a widespread grassroots effort to try to weave the principles of social justice into the fabric of the American psyche. A more fruitful approach might be to convince the Gang of Four to voluntarily dismantle the windmills, to make them see that it would be to the advantage of not only the American people, but also in their own economic interest, to embrace universal coverage.

Seemingly, it would be difficult to convince the insurance companies to (in effect) self-destruct. It could mean shutting their doors and laying off many of their 1.3 million employees. Yet, as the cost of health care increases exponentially and health insurance becomes increasingly unaffordable, insurance companies may want to get out of "risk" situations in health care. They could shift their role and become contract administrators for a national health plan. They would get their cut of the payments. And they could avoid potential losses, the kinds of losses suffered by about half of the for-profit HMOs in the waning days of the managed-care bubble. They could voluntarily choose to get out of the "risk" business.

The Drug Barons

THE PHARMACEUTICAL COMPANIES WILL FIGHT fiercely to defend their windmills. They owe it to their stockholders. However, under pressure, they have been retreating in a few areas. On the international front, they reduced their prices on drugs used for HIV/AIDS. They even offered to donate the drugs. But their capitulation only came after years of maintaining high prices for everyone. They gave in only when it was apparent that cheaper generic versions of the drugs would come from India or Brazil. The drug companies have tried to sweeten their own image with charity-type programs in the United States, like Pfizer's "Sharing the Care" program in community health centers, including ours. Pfizer and other pharmaceutical companies have now come out with a low-cost (in Pfizer's case, $15 a drug) prescription offer for low-income Americans—likely a response to the hullabaloo raised by windmill chasers. These programs do help low-income people, and they cost the drug companies almost nothing. The people affected would have been unable to afford the medicines anyway. Meanwhile, the pharmaceutical companies earn brand loyalty from the clinicians who prescribe their drugs.

In the big picture, the pharmaceutical industry will fight to retain its profits since that is their primary mission. Some analysts argue that if we had national health insurance (NHI), the drug companies' profits wouldn't necessarily drop. They would in theory make up in volume what they lose by cutting prices. In the long run, the United States will undoubtedly adopt price controls for drugs, just as every other developed country has done. At some point, our leaders will realize that it is in the greater interest of our nation to have access to effective and affordable care than to sustain a specific industry at a rate of profit margin way in excess of any other industry.

The rhetoric that (1) the pharmaceutical industry needs its huge profit margin for research and development, and that (2) drugs have to be more expensive in the United States because American companies do the lion's share of developing new drugs is myth and rubbish (see Chapter 1, Myth #11). They've got a good deal going, and who can blame them for wanting to keep it working for them? They will fight the battle to maximize their profits until they see the writing on the wall that says "price controls." Maybe then they will voluntarily come over to the side of NHI.

The Camelots of Health Care

DESPITE THE RECENT PROLIFERATION of for-profit hospitals, most hospitals have the interest of their communities in mind. But the field of inpatient care has changed in recent years. It has become a much more diverse entity. Nursing homes, which used to be mostly community-based, have now largely been converted to for-profit, chain ownership. Much of what used to be done as inpatient care has now been converted to outpatient care at ambulatory care centers. These have been largely for-profit entities. They attract the paying patients and procedures. Thus, they have left the hospitals with a greater share of the uncompensated care. And the hospitals cannot turn away (or refuse to admit) patients who walk into their ERs—including the uninsured. From a fiscal standpoint, the hospitals should support NHI.

Unfortunately, the hospitals' experience with Medicare has often been unfavorable and frustrating. When I advocate for an improved and expanded Medicare for All, many hospital administrators roll their eyes. They've been so stressed out with dealing with Medicare's bureaucratic demands that they worry about having more of "such a good thing." Depending on their Medicare/managed-care mix, hospitals may in alternate years complain about how their private-sector payments must subsidize Medicare, or vice versa. But they will admit that the managed-care bureaucratic burdens are often worse than Medicare's. And the prospect of having only one insurance payer with one set of forms and rules does provide a measure of hope for the hospitals. Their administrative burdens could be vastly simplified.

In the old days, Medicare just paid the hospital's bill, no strings attached. But since the initiation of DRGs (Diagnosis Related Groups, or where Medicare pays a hospital by diagnosis, no matter how long the patient stays in the hospital), and other bureaucratic demands, hospitals have been much more wary of Medicare. The hospitals, especially the for-profits, brought much of this added red tape on themselves. Medicare fraud, like the fraudulent up-coding done systematically by HCA/Columbia, precipitated the tightening of the screws. "Improving" Medicare means making it simpler. But we also need to expect a greater degree of honesty on the part of health care providers. This honesty will be difficult to achieve without removing incentives to maximize shareholder profits. The for-profits will be difficult to convince. Maybe they should be converted to a not-for-profit status so we once again have "a level playing field" in health care. Not-for-profit hospitals should have every reason to support NHI since they would no longer have to write off their services to uninsured patients as uncompensated care.

The Lords of Medicine

THE PHYSICIANS ARE A mixed bag. A large number of physicians of all specialties (especially primary care doctors and psychiatrists) actually support single-payer universal coverage. Physicians for a National Health Program (PNHP), an organization started in 1987 to promote single-payer national health insurance, has more than 14,000 members, and its ranks are growing daily. However, many physicians underestimate how much their colleagues support NHI, as a recent study showed. In a national survey of medical school faculty, residents and students, published in the *New England Journal of Medicine* in 1999, 57 percent chose single payer as the best solution for America's health care ills.[3] However, the medical establishment, as represented by the American Medical Association (AMA), has been staunchly against single-payer universal coverage. Fearing a Canadian-style health care system, the AMA spent millions of dollars in the early '90s to finance an advertising campaign of disinformation aimed at discrediting Canada's system of universal coverage. The AMA prefers system changes that, bluntly described, would protect and increase physicians' income and autonomy. Their solution stresses "personal responsibility" and patient "choice" (with the physician still in the driver's seat) through constructs such as health savings accounts (HSAs) and tax credits.

It amazes me how generally ignorant many, if not most, physicians are about how our health care system works—or doesn't work. Some may be motivated by their own narrow economic interests, but many do care about improving access to health care. Yet they have no idea of the larger picture, especially from their patients' viewpoint. Despite spending long hours buried in the everyday work of their profession, most physicians remain "technicians." They have little appreciation of the difficulties faced by the uninsured and (now) underinsured. They are simply too busy, too tied up in their daily chaos, to take notice of what is really happening to their patients. More poignantly, they are even more unaware of the patients they never see. Those are the uninsured patients who (1) come in but aren't seen because they lack the $200 they're asked to plunk down at the front desk, or (2) don't even bother to come in because they don't have the cash in hand and have too much pride to be rebuffed by the receptionist.

The physicians—as well as other health care professionals—should be much easier to convince to tear down the windmills. In fact, many professional organizations have been actively coming up with proposals for universal coverage, some of them quite progressive (beyond such narrow solutions as HSAs). Some of the proposed plans have even been really "universal," such as the proposal being put forward by the American Academy of Family Physicians (AAFP). Their plan calls for (in effect) single-payer universal coverage for primary care, prevention, and catastrophic costs. Their original draft even excluded deductibles and co-payments, though they reinstated the co-payments in the final version. The AAFP plan advocates tax-based financing as well as separation of employers from the purchasing of health insurance. What a long way physicians have come.

It remains unlikely that the Mother of all American medical associations (the AMA), with its long history of largely successful opposition to national health insurance—they helped derail every plan in the twentieth century—will support any meaningful solution. But the AMA is losing its influence as the other medical organizations take leadership on this vital issue. There is hope.

Physicians are increasingly discussing universal coverage. It's only a matter of time until they realize the need for an affordable, equitable solution that embraces national health insurance.

Tilting at Windmills From Beyond the Medical Establishment

THERE ARE OPPORTUNITIES outside the Gang of Four to do battle with the windmills. Perhaps the most promising hope for action comes from convincing the American business community that national health insurance (NHI) would be in their economic self-interest (see Chapter 3). It's evident that NHI would also be in the best interest of their employees. It would be a way to break the perverse and increasingly onerous link between employment and health insurance. The link developed as a fluke of history. During World War II wage controls froze workers' pay, so employers began to offer employees health insurance as an extra benefit. No other developed country has this anachronistic mechanism. Nonetheless, recent surveys show that a large majority of the American public is satisfied with the employer-based system. Perhaps the respondents were unaware of other options, but their comfort with the current system illustrates how difficult it may be to convince Americans that a change would be to their advantage.

The time is quickly approaching, however, when business will have to take a hard look at how it is providing health insurance for employees. The impetus behind the managed-care revolution of a decade ago came from business. Under economic siege from rapidly escalating health insurance costs, business led the change to managed-care plans to control runaway costs. The "fix" was temporary, and health insurance costs are again increasing at double-digit rates. Employers have already been shifting costs to employees with ever-increasing co-pays and deductibles. And employees are starting to hurt more as they join the swelling ranks of the "underinsured." Now employers are looking toward HSAs and "defined-contribution" approaches, euphemisms for further shifting the costs to employees. The effect would be to cut loose the employees' security lines in a wild sea of increasing premiums for health insurance.

For a while, not so long ago when the unemployment rate was low, some employers regarded the health insurance benefit as a recruitment and retention tool. But with a rising unemployment rate, this factor is no longer so important. Employers are likely to wake up soon, see the light at the end of the tunnel, and shed their health insurance relationship with their employees. It makes economic sense—especially in a global market where competing corporations in other nations are not saddled with this albatross of a cost. Employees will experience a progressively more difficult time in navigating an increasingly expensive and perilous health insurance market. If they should be so unfortunate as to have a preexisting condition, they will be even worse off. The obvious affordable and practical solution would be automatic universal coverage with a single risk pool. Business has to wake up soon, if for no other reason than out of economic self-interest. And when business speaks, America and American politicians listen.

There are new opportunities for windmill bashing since 9/11. Compared to a sense of community, "personal responsibility"— everyone for himself—doesn't seem to be quite as important as it used to be. Out of the disaster has come a feeling that we're a community, that we have some shared responsibility for each other. Even "government" seems to have gained some stature. In an October 2001 *New York Times* op-ed piece, Robert Putnam, author of *Bowling Alone: The Collapse and Revival of American Community,* opined that the new sense of community would not be short-lived. He concluded that, "This new period of crisis can make real to us and our children the value of deeper community connections."[4] In addition, there's the whole new dilemma of what we do for victims of bioterrorism. A special fund? New complex eligibility rules to access the fund? Everyone for himself? Out of 9/11, there's new hope for universal coverage. The "we're all in this together" argument has a new validity that more Americans can now appreciate.

If we can pull together enough Don Quixotes, we can create a large enough grassroots movement to demand change because "we're all in this together." As an inveterate Don Q. myself, I'd like to deputize every man, woman, and child in America for the cause. Maybe then the medical-industrial complex would be forced to capitulate, to realize that the interests of America as a whole will be better served if we have universal coverage. And, as a true dreamer, I'm campaigning for 100 percent, not 92 or 95 percent, because the forgotten 5 or 8 percent are bound to be my patients. They're the ones most likely to fall between the cracks because (1) they don't have the means to negotiate a ridiculously complex system, or (2) they have conditions that make them health insurance pariahs.

Most thoughtful people, including business and corporate gurus, who have lived with our dysfunctional nonsystem for decades, admit that America eventually will have to go to some type of national health insurance. Many even use the words "single payer." The windmills will fall. I hope it will be sooner rather than later. The sooner it comes, the less the disenfranchised—those without adequate access to timely care—will have to suffer needless anguish and misery. Meanwhile, we are likely to pursue a variety of partial fixes or piecemeal approaches as we attempt to find "a uniquely American" solution. Doc Quixote will realize his dream—some day. And it will take a grassroots approach to get there.

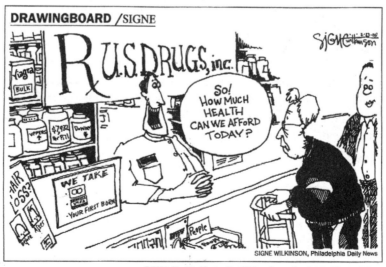

© 2000, The Washington Post Writers Group. Reprinted with permission.

Summary of Key Points

- It's likely that some sectors of the medical-industrial complex will see an advantage to universal coverage with national health insurance. Undoubtedly, some will not, and the struggle will not be easy.

- As they have become more informed, physicians have increasingly become more favorably disposed toward universal coverage.

- Businesses need to wake up and realize that their current role in purchasing health insurance is not only outdated but also puts them at a competitive disadvantage with their counterparts in other countries.

- It will take a grassroots effort to change our system, but the system will change eventually.

Chapter 13

In Search of a "Uniquely American" Solution to Health Care for All

"We need a pragmatic, not an ideological, solution. Reduce the number [of uninsured Americans] from 39 million to its irreducible minimum, probably about 15 million, and consider that a victory and not a terrible tragedy."

—Dr. Richard Corlin, president of the AMA, speaking in Cedar Rapids, IA, April 2002[1]

IN MY WORK AS A PHYSICIAN at a "safety-net" clinic, I am aware on a daily basis of the problems faced by the uninsured and, now increasingly, the underinsured.

The conventional wisdom of our health industry gurus and our political leaders tells us that, to solve our uniquely American problems with health care, we will need a uniquely American solution. Of course, we are already unique in many ways. We're the only developed country without universal coverage. We're unique in how we so closely tie health insurance to employment. We're unique in having such a high proportion of personal bankruptcies—almost 50 percent—tied to medical bills. We also may be unique in our ability to get so little value for the huge amount of money we spend on health care. British, French, Cuban, or Canadian solutions will not do.

The issues are complex. Health care organization is not simple. Multiple solutions proposed over the past 90 years have been shot down,[2] deemed either impossible, unworkable, overly bureaucratic, too dependent on government, too expensive, or simply unacceptable to the American public.

Unfortunately, the direction we appear to be headed could lead to "health care meltdown." We're becoming more of a multitiered system that progressively excludes the poor and the sick, and soon (if not already) the middle class as well. Piecemeal approaches with increased complexity—such as tax credits, vouchers, "defined contributions" with managed care and health savings accounts (HSAs)—will only result in more holes for people to fall through, more delayed care. A few may benefit, but many will be harmed. Why not consider simplifying the system?

Perhaps we need to "think outside of the box," consider an alternative, which should garner support as the antithesis of "socialized medicine." Why not consider an approach that would maximize the American value of "personal responsibility," level the playing field, and be truly universal in nature? How about considering, as an intellectual exercise, an approach that reflects the logical (and absurd) endpoint of present-day conservative thinking in America, a "uniquely American" solution: universal uninsurance?

Universal Uninsurance

DO AWAY WITH ALL health insurance. Abolish it completely. Allow free exercise of our ability to be creative and entrepreneurial. We could remold our health care system using the American values of rugged individualism, personal responsibility, belief in the free market, and—not to be forgotten—compassion for our neighbors.

Eliminating bureaucracies like Medicare, Medicaid, HMOs, and health insurance companies would save billions of dollars. Employers would be relieved of the burden of providing health insurance for their workers. Employees would get larger paychecks instead of having their hard-earned wages diverted to ever more expensive health insurance plans with increasingly shrinking benefits. People would be forced to care about the cost of their health care. Managed care would be gone. No longer would we have messy, unfair, and resource-wasting government regulations or restraints on utilization and referrals. Two hours on the phone to get a procedure approved?

American technology would form part of the solution. Consumers would be incentivized to make much greater use of the Internet for health information. In true American style we could have huge health care mega-malls, like Wal-Health or Health Depot. Shopping centers could offer a wide range of practitioners, including alternative medicine. Blue light specials. Coupons to clip in the Sunday papers for discounts on colon cancer screening. Half-price purple pills (flown in from Mexico). The possibilities are limitless.

What About Poor Folks?
Charity Care to the Rescue

BUT WHAT WOULD HAPPEN to poor folks? The people without even enough money to buy the Sunday paper to clip the coupons? Or the homeless folks without a mailing address to receive the junk mail with money-saving health care specials?

We will look to our past and the great American tradition of charity care. Physicians who are nostalgia buffs will be overjoyed to be able once again to offer free care to the needy. Freed up from the bare-bones payments of managed-care plans and Medicaid, physicians will be able to afford giving charity care. Hospitals will again have the capacity to cost shift.

Compassion could flourish. After all, compassion, as in "compassionate conservatism," is part of the American way of being. Poor folks will once again be able to feel grateful for the free or reduced-price care they receive. It will be individuals helping individuals, not the government butting in. We will be able to circumvent the whole messy philosophic argument about health care being a human right.

There could be a profusion of free clinics. The plethora of bored specialists who retired early to escape managed care could volunteer to work in free clinics. For people too proud to use the services of free clinics, but still unable to afford needed health care, there could be a host of pluralistic solutions for financing their care. Americans love pluralistic solutions—and choice—or so we're told.

Some tried-and-true American solutions for financing health care for individuals in need:

- The bake sale. Selling only 1,000 three-layer chocolate cakes at $8.99 each could finance a gallbladder operation, if the beneficiary only stayed in the hospital one day. For those who might be interested in extending this model on a nationwide scale, if each person in America sold just one 9-inch German chocolate cake a day at $9.99 apiece, the proceeds ($1 trillion) would be enough to cover 100 percent of America's health care costs, assuming administrative savings from eliminating insurance. There would also be a grand opportunity for choice/pluralism: we could sell apple pies, peach cobblers, cherry cheesecakes, etc. The possibilities are limitless.

Health Care Financing – and Choice – U.S. Style

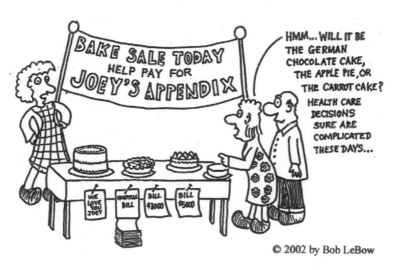

© 2002 by Bob LeBow

- Coin boxes at supermarket checkout stands and self-service gas stations to collect money for, say, Sammy's hernia repair, or Max's Viagra.

- Lotteries or bingo games set up on an *ad hoc* basis to meet the crisis health care needs of a needy individual.

- To raise money for expensive procedures, an array of other activities, such as concerts, telethons, phone cards, car washes, donating the cost of a meal not eaten, mowing lawns, etc. (Columnist Molly Ivins relates "There are more than 1,000 concerts given every week by musicians for other musicians to raise money for an operation or medical treatment of some kind.")[3]

These types of activities, like holding a raffle to pay for an emergency appendectomy, provide great opportunities for building cohesiveness in a community. In fact, if communities elect to go even further, they could come up with community-based approaches to health care financing. Catastrophic funds, hospital taxing districts, local sales taxes for health, sin taxes, and the use of tobacco funds are but a few of the innovative ways in which communities could respond to the need. Charitable foundations and religious organizations could supplement these funds.

Perhaps the most attractive aspect of universal uninsurance is the level to which it raises the importance of "personal responsibility." It's almost like the TV game of "Survival."

Potential Obstacles to Universal Uninsurance

WHAT ABOUT PEOPLE WITH Medicare? Wouldn't they oppose this approach? Most would probably support the change once they realized that Medicare is in fact a government program. Others would need to be convinced that it was the American way, that it wasn't proper for America to have a health care system that looked anything like those other countries' socialized medicine.

And what about people who might be inclined to buy insurance to protect themselves from financial ruin? The nonbelievers who are skeptical of "bake-sale" financing? They would need to be convinced that their sentiments were un-American, perhaps even unpatriotic. They would need to renew their faith in "the market."

Of course, it's unlikely that pure universal uninsurance could ever become a reality in America. As a colleague told me, Americans are hesitant to support "one size fits all." Even more significantly, the insurance companies, hospitals, and pharmaceutical industry would all oppose it. Demand could evaporate for the $1,000 toenail fungus treatment that people read about in the Sunday supplements. They could no longer demand the product "because their insurance paid for it." Sales of $80 a month Clarinex might drop when people realized they could buy a generic drug with equivalent efficacy for $2 a month. And health insurers would obviously be out of business. Employers might even oppose it, as employees would likely have more freedom to change jobs, just as they would with the diametrically opposite approach to health care reform, national health insurance.

The Sad Truth: Fantasy May Resemble Reality

IT'S UNCANNY, however, how much this tongue-in-cheek spoof I have described on universal uninsurance resembles reality. It's a direction in which American health care could be headed. A game of "Survival"—even for the middle class. There are even some people, like the members of a basically libertarian organization called the American Association of Physicians and Surgeons, who could actually support the universal uninsurance fantasy as I've described it.

The newest maneuvers *du jour* to control costs (for employers, but not employees) are scary in their resemblance to universal uninsurance. Business interests seem to be heading in the direction of a "defined-contribution" approach. This strategy in effect caps employer spending for health insurance and shifts costs— and risk—to employees. It's like the model outlined above with a fixed employer contribution thrown in. For someone who has a chronic illness or who gets sick or is injured, "defined contribution" is like a crapshoot. And it does nothing to address the problem of the uninsured.

Promoters of the "defined-contribution" approach have dressed up the idea by terming it "consumer-driven" health care, when it's really "risk-assumed-by-employee" health care.

Extolling the myth of "more choice," and they don't really mean it, the plan cuts employees loose in a market of rapidly escalating health care costs. Those with limited funds will suffer as they are left to navigate for themselves in a market that is complex and confusing. The Internet, advocated by the proponents of "defined contributions" as a tool to educate consumers, is grossly over-estimated in its usefulness. It's still a tool in its infancy, even for providers. The modern-day snake oil merchants, selling their expensive and sometimes marginally effective health care prod-ucts and insurance, will retain their advantage.

Insurance companies are scrambling to design a variety of "defined-contribution" options for business. Once again we have vested interests, at least the insurance companies and employers, heading toward an option that places the interest of sick patients last. Many conservatives and physician groups, meanwhile, support close relatives of the "defined-contribution" approach: health savings accounts, vouchers, and tax credits.

At some point, we Americans will have to wake up. Perhaps our attachment to the mantra of "personal responsibility" and "the market" is so strong that we would actually support a solu-tion under which some people can get PET scans, others leeches. Or maybe it's okay with us if low-income folks get a ten-dollar 991-minute phone card to talk to Dial-a-Nurse in Bangalore while wealthier Americans buy "concierge care" and have their own private physicians. Hopefully, that kind of approach, or the reliance on bake-sale financing, will not be the "uniquely American" solution we choose. But while we're in health care "limbo," variations on the status quo will see us head in that very direction. And, meanwhile, the vested interests will continue to reap their profits since they hold the advantage in a game of "Survivor."

Maybe we need to reconsider our insistence on a "uniquely American" solution. Perhaps we need to wake up, accept the obvious, put aside the myths, learn from the experience of other countries, and adopt a system based on "one risk pool" that gives every person in America affordable and accessible health care. Perhaps, as the famous Winston Churchill quote goes, we Americans are destined to try every other system first (including maybe even universal uninsurance), before we do the right thing.

Summary of Key Points

- America's health care financing system is unfair, illogical, costly, chaotic, confusing, absurd, and at times laughable.

- Our health care financing system is currently in danger of becoming even more complex and chaotic with some of the newer proposals (such as tax credits and vouchers) for "reducing the number of uninsured."

- We are headed toward a multitiered health care system in the United States—a system in which an increasing number of Americans (including many middle-class people) will be forced to play a game of "Survivor."

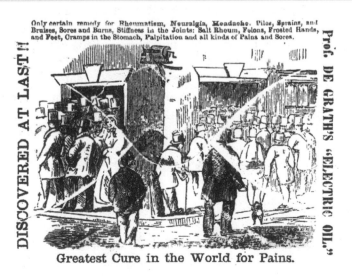

Only certain remedy for Rheumatism, Neuralgia, Headache. Piles, Sprains, and Bruises, Sores and Burns, Stiffness in the Joints: Salt Rheum, Felons, Frosted Hands, and Feet, Cramps in the Stomach, Palpitation and all kinds of Pains and Sores.

DISCOVERED AT LAST!!

Prof. DE GRATH'S "ELECTRIC OIL."

Greatest Cure in the World for Pains.

Chapter 14

Grassroots for Health Care for All: What Can Americans Do to Claim a Right to Health Care?

I have a fantasy. I see a huge football stadium full of people. Cheerleaders are leading the crowd: "Give me an H . . . ." People in the stands turn over placards, one at a time. Finally, all the cards are up. They read "HEALTH CARE FOR ALL," and the crowd stomps and roars with approval.

I RECENTLY DID A PERSONAL MINI-SURVEY of the patients at my clinic. I asked why they thought the United States, as opposed to all the other developed nations, did not guarantee health insurance to all its citizens. I got an interesting array of answers (see Chapter 5). Many replied, at least initially, that they didn't know why, or that "we couldn't afford it." But one 62-year-old woman asserted, "We need to unite, get together, and demand universal coverage."

It's difficult to get large numbers of people interested in health care reform, let alone become activists. Discussions on health policy, if they go on for over a few minutes, more often than not get a glazed-eye response. Yet, without major popular support, without that stadium full of cheering people, movement toward any substantial reform—let alone a sweeping change such as national health insurance—will most likely remain a dream. Our political system makes this kind of fundamental change a daunting task. There are many other factors that also work against our efforts, including:

- The public's general lack of knowledge on the issue.

- Automatic prejudices, in the form of doubt-provoking sound bites, that have become a part of Americans' subconscious thinking. These attitudes have been created and reinforced by years of misinformation and myths.

- Politically and financially powerful corporate and medical interests (and their lobbyists and money), which are committed to stymie any efforts at change.

- A culture that generally believes in "market" solutions, individualism, and a "bootstrap" mentality, as opposed to health care as a basic human right.

- Habit. People are generally accepting of what they are accustomed to and fearful of change.

- A sense of security in the status quo for those Americans who are relatively well-off, a security that could somehow be threatened or lessened by change.

- No personal bad experience with the system by most people, especially middle-class insured people, at least up to now. They have been fairly well and have not had to use the system for any significant services.

- People not "hurting enough" to get personally involved.

- Apathy. People, including physicians, are tied up in the hectic activities of their daily lives.

- No sense of community. Despite 9/11, Americans are not community-oriented people. Most Americans are more motivated to put the interests of the individual or the family first.

- The appearance that "something" is already being done. Incremental or piecemeal actions such as SCHIP or "patient protection" acts may defuse some of the demand for action.

- Similarly, the high level of "lip service" to universal coverage with an array of complex and ineffectual proposals (but not national health insurance or Medicare for All). This activity creates the impression that there is motion toward change.

- Lack of adequate financial support. The whole movement toward universal coverage through national health insurance (NHI) lacks adequate financial support, as opposed to the well-heeled forces arrayed against NHI.

- Disenfranchisement of the uninsured. As a group, they are largely politically disenfranchised and lack lobbyists or political clout.

- Failure of activists to agree upon a unified strategy or action plan to reach Health Care for All.

Facing these seemingly insurmountable obstacles, what steps can we take to create a groundswell of public support for Health Care for All?

Timing and the Changing Battlefield

IN NOVEMBER 2001, the National Council on Health Care came out with an essay, "A Perfect Storm," by Joel Miller.[1] In this treatise, Miller postulates that there will soon be a convergence of the proper conditions to create an overwhelming public demand for universal coverage—akin to the weather conditions that made the "Perfect Storm" in the movie by that name. The principal converging factors: (1) a rapidly increasing number of uninsured and underinsured; (2) a marked rise in health insurance premiums and the cost of health care; (3) a worsening economy (which may be temporary, but will likely affect low-income people more); (4) a growing number of unemployed people; and (5) a demand for relief from employers. With all of the above conditions, state governments, which are already facing soaring expenditures for the Medicaid safety net, are likely to reach a state of fiscal panic.

Like the Taliban facing crisis conditions, the players on the health care battlefield could switch sides, even peaceably (see Chapter 12). Employers could demand relief and ask the government to take responsibility for insuring everyone. States will likely ask for a higher federal match for Medicaid. Harry and Louise could see the light, "get religion," realize there is a better way, and join the forces for universal coverage—maybe even national health insurance or an improved Medicare for All.

The corporate side will, of course, develop new strategies and permutations of the same old games to maximize the time they have to reap profits—in the same manner in which the pharmaceutical companies game the system to extend their patents. Universal coverage will continue to get lip service from all. There will be more "summits" to create the image that the elite care and are doing something to promote change. I personally won't believe they're serious about doing anything more than wringing the last dollar they can possibly squeeze out of the system until they put their money where their words are. Instead of seeing a $60 million ad campaign about the "bus from Canada," I'd like to see the drug companies, the insurance industry, and the AMA pool their resources on a $60 million publicity effort to persuade Americans to support national health insurance. It wouldn't be so impossible if business joined the bandwagon.

Timing is key. If the "Perfect Storm" should happen—and past forecasts of both weather and health care crises have been known to be fickle—then the grassroots support should be there to assure that the corporate guys can't pull off another shell game. The medical-industrial complex is not to be trusted. It can be held accountable if an informed and "hurting" public can be mobilized at the right time to fight for meaningful Health Care for All.

What do we Americans need to do to take advantage of the right moment, the magic hour when the stars are aligned just properly for health care reform? How can we be ready to "scramble" when the opportunity appears? Political winds can shift quickly, and openings for action can happen suddenly and disappear just as fast. We need to be prepared. If we're not ready, we could well wait another decade for the next opening. Realists would argue that, given the present administration in Washington, a reform as radical as national health insurance has about as much chance of passing as a snowball in hell. The Bush administration, if anything, has been promoting exactly the opposite: privatizing and/or dismembering Medicare—as well as Social Security. But

2008 is not far away. Already it appears there has been a prominent defector from the pro-privatization forces. In a campaign speech in Louisiana, Senator John Breaux (D-LA), who only a short while ago was promoting the privatization of Medicare, came out and said, "You ought to have health care as a basic right. Everybody in America should have health insurance and we should help people get it."[2] Politics acts in strange ways.

Groups, Old and New, Promoting Health Care for All

THE *WALL STREET JOURNAL* ran a front-page article on December 17, 2001, by Ron Winslow in which he talked about a rash of new organizations—he termed them "the sons of Jackson Hole"—that are working on solutions to our health care mess. Most of these didn't seem to be promoting Health Care for All. But a few new groups, like America's Health Together, are.

There are many other groups and/or coalitions that have been actively promoting universal coverage for years. Studying our health care system and the uninsured has been a major activity for some of these organizations, like the National Council on Health Care, which is comprised predominantly of major corporations. Education of the public has been a priority, although the degree of the public's knowledge so far has not been particularly impressive. Some foundations, like the Kaiser Family Foundation, have been cranking out useful information without endorsing a specific solution. Others, like the Commonwealth Fund, have financed numerous studies on the uninsured—and have also come up with specific proposals. One such plan came from Families USA, which joined with the Health Insurance Association of America (HIAA) to come up with the so-called "strange bedfellows" proposal for universal coverage.

On February 12, 2002, a day after President Bush's airing of his plans for health care, a group of 13 national organizations, led by the Robert Wood Johnson Foundation, came out with a new initiative that they named "CoveringTheUninsured."[3] They announced a $10 million television and print advertising campaign to publicize the plight of the uninsured. Part of their efforts are laudable, such as educating the American public about the obstacles faced by the uninsured or pointing out that 8 out of 10 uninsured Americans are in working families. Unfortunately, their initiative falls far short of what is needed. It may even signal a retreat from previous efforts that advocated for "universal coverage." In "seek[ing] solutions to the problem of the uninsured," they speak only of "reducing the number of the uninsured." They are clearly endorsing an "incremental" strategy, not universal coverage. One of its supporters rejected the single-payer approach as unaffordable. And only one of the sponsors, the Catholic Health Association, represented by Michael Collins, MD, came out and specifically stated that *all Americans* should be afforded the justice of getting health care coverage, although John Sweeney, president of the AFL-CIO, did allude to "covering every American."

There is a general recognition that the American public has a woefully poor knowledge of what's happening in health care. The issues are difficult to explain because they are complex, confusing, and often politically charged. Physicians for a National Health Program (PNHP) has been striving over the past 15 years to educate primarily physicians but also others. PNHP uses hard data to show how America would benefit from national health insurance. PNHP researchers have also been documenting with studies how our system has been exploited and (literally) pillaged by investor-owned for-profit health care.

The public health community has been strongly supportive of Health Care for All. Medical groups such as the American Academy of Family Practice (AAFP) have laboriously developed proposals for universal coverage. The AAFP went so far as to propose truly universal coverage (everybody in) for primary care and prevention, with a publicly administered system that abolishes the employer link and has tax-based financing. The ACP-ASIM (the internal medicine specialists) actually spent a million dollars to buy ads promoting universal coverage. And in April 2002, they came out with a stepwise (over 7 years) proposal that would provide health insurance coverage for every American. Their proposal is based on the expansion of Medicaid and SCHIP plus premium support, so it fails to address the issue of affordability and leaves our fragmented, overly complex, and wasteful system intact. At least they're sincere in their efforts. A few professional groups, like the American Nurses Association (ANA) and the American Medical Student Association (AMSA), have been solid national health insurance supporters for years.

The Community-Based Efforts

IN ADDITION TO THE professional groups that are pushing for health care reform and universal coverage, there are many community-based groups that are fighting for Health Care for All at the state level. In fact, many state Legislatures working with these groups have started to formulate their own unique solutions to universal coverage, convinced that no meaningful solutions will be seen on a federal level, at least not in the foreseeable future.

In November 2001, voters in Portland, Maine, passed a non-binding referendum endorsing single-payer universal coverage despite being vastly outspent by the opposition. Anthem Blue Shield, a for-profit insurer (and the largest insurer in Maine), spent nearly $400,000 on advertising in the last 2 weeks before the vote in an attempt to convince the voters to reject the referendum. The supporters of single-payer universal coverage only had about $15,000 to spend, but they won. Their victory inspired speculation that the time was propitious for a new national debate on health care.[4]

In 2006, ten states introduced bills that specified some form of universal coverage. Most of these bills did not even get out of committee. However, Massachusetts and Vermont did pass legislation as an attempt to provide health insurance for all their citizens. The one that seemed to create the most press was the Health Care Access and Affordability Act from Massachusetts. This bill attempts to address inadequate access to health care through a combination of public and private funding. It mandates that everyone who can afford health insurance, either through a state-run program or private insurance, must buy it. It will expand the state Medicaid program and require that all businesses with ten or more employees offer health insurance to their workforce or be fined $295 per employee. It encourages insurance companies to expand their options for low-cost plans and offers an increase in Medicaid reimbursement to certain providers.

What a political coup! Finally, a health care reform act that was found to be politically feasible. If the reader has been paying attention thus far, he or she has probably formed a few opinions and is already asking several questions like: "How in the world is this program going to fix health care in Massachusetts?" We will expound on that in the Conclusion section. Let's see if we both come to similar conclusions. In the meantime, suffice it to say that public policy is frequently driven by three motivating factors: fear, ignorance, and greed or self- interest. The astute reader will find evidence of all three in the Massachusetts bill.

Recently, the Health Resources Service Administration (HRSA), part of Health and Human Services (HHS), gave about a million dollars to each of 20 states to study the problems of the uninsured in their respective states and to come up with some options for decreasing the numbers of the uninsured. The grants' stated purpose was actually to promote getting insurance coverage for "all," but the "all" got diluted in practice. However, at least in Idaho, and I'm sure in other states as well, the grant served the purpose of helping to educate health care leaders and legislators (and the public, though to a much lesser degree) on the issues surrounding the uninsured. Idaho's legislators, for example, were surprised to learn that 80 percent of the uninsured were people in working families. And useful studies came out of the HRSA grants, like the cost analyses of single-payer universal coverage that were done in Vermont and California. Both showed that the single-payer approach would not only cover everyone, but it would also save 5 percent overall.

At the Congressional level, there has been some simmering activity to try to lay the groundwork for Health Care for All—and promise of some real action in the near future. So far, there has been little current support for broad proposals, like Bill Clinton's ill-fated "Managed Competition for All" plan or Jim McDermott's (D-WA) HR 1200. The latter had at one point garnered 140 cosponsors for single-payer universal coverage. But there has been talk of bills to facilitate state-by-state single-payer efforts as well as to provide waivers so the federal programs can be included in a state's single-payer plan. And in February 2003, John Conyers (D-MI) introduced the United States National Health Insurance Act (HR 676), which is basically a "Medicare for All" and is gaining support across the nation. The bill can be read in its entirety and further discussion of its virtues can be found at <www.pnhp.org>.

Meanwhile, there has been a movement to gain support for universal coverage through House Concurrent Resolution (HCR) 99. This resolution, also called the "Health Care Access Resolution," lists and endorses all the positive features of Health Care for All, but it avoids mentioning any specific approach. Its supporters, which include many activist organizations, seem to be trying to stay on politically safe ground so they can garner more general support for universal coverage itself. It's unclear if the proponents of HCR 99 are laying the groundwork to build general support for what will become national health insurance. Yet it's hard to imagine that the principles outlined in the resolution, if implemented, could be anything but a national health insurance solution. Some of the backers of HCR 99, however, may have given up on a truly comprehensive solution and may be seeking "the best they can get" for the American people. An April 30, 2002, panel discussion of HCR 99 can be viewed at <www.kff.org>, the Web site of the Kaiser Family Foundation.

On the Internet, there are now a host of Web sites that disseminate useful information about our health care system and its problems, including <www.pnhp.org>, <www.cmwf.org>, <www.kff.org>, and <www.everybodyinnobodyout.org>, to mention but a few.

More Talk, Less Progress?

DESPITE ALL THE EFFORTS of these groups to raise America's consciousness of our problems with health care, there continues to be a very high level of cluelessness at all levels, from the general public to our leaders, and even health care professionals. There also is a worrisome level of disagreement among activist groups about strategy. Some would describe the split as one between pragmatists and idealists. Only 2 or 3 years ago, there seemed to be some strong consensus for a single-payer solution, like an improved Medicare for All. But, perhaps out of frustration or impatience—or pragmatism—many former single-payer advocates, like UHCAN (Universal Health Coverage for America Network), modified their demand for national health insurance. Some past supporters of the single-payer approach have gone so far as to assert, "If you insist on holding out for single payer, you'll get nothing!" In a September 27, 2001, MSNBC editorial, University of Pennsylvania bioethicist Art Caplan took that position (see Chapter 16).

In the everyday real world of health care, all of us who work with health get involved with so-called "incremental" actions. We try to qualify people for Medicaid. We lobby so that SCHIP funding will not be cut. We volunteer at free clinics. We fight to get support for Critical Access Hospitals. Some health care activists argue for doing absolutely nothing—so that the whole system will implode sooner. But being the compassionate people we are, the nihilist ("tough love") approach is hard to accept when we see so much injustice and need. How can we stand by and do nothing tangible? The collective mission of grassroots activists should be to remind each other (in the words of Darth Vader) to "keep our eye on the leader"—to maintain the vision. The ultimate goal ("leader") is universal coverage that is affordable, comprehensive, and equitable.

Meanwhile, we fight the daily skirmishes—because we have to—while keeping our eye on the prize. It is unfortunate that activist groups cannot be more united in their strategies and messages. As time passes, however, the level of consciousness should increase. When that rising level of consciousness meets an escalating level of "public pain," the time will be ripe for meaningful reform—assuming a few more stars, like the political will, are lined up correctly. We should hold steady on our goal of national health insurance, but it may well require a "next best step" strategy, like stepwise expansion of Medicare or a state-by-state approach to get the process rolling.

What Specific Action Steps Will It Take to Motivate Grassroots America?

AS HAS BEEN BRIEFLY OUTLINED ABOVE, an impressive amount of groundwork has already been done at many levels to create an infrastructure that can be used to promote Health Care for All in America. But because the issue is so complex and confusing, it's relatively easy for the well-heeled opponents of meaningful health care reform to derail progress towards a solution such as national health insurance. All they need to do to obstruct change is create doubt among the public and our political leaders. To effect their negative objectives, they have huge financial resources. And they have access to the politicians, access they have facilitated through campaign contributions.

Given the power of the medical-industrial complex, what can be done, what specific action steps can activists take to win over the hearts and souls of grassroots America? How can we get ordinary Americans to support Health Care for All? Part of the answer must come from addressing the problem areas outlined at the beginning of this chapter. In brief, some likely (and practical) steps would be:

- Develop, with the help of publicists, a series of simple, to the point, targeted messages[5] to change how people respond to Health Care for All and to counter the gut-level sound bites that stop the conversation. We are selling a good product. The opposition is selling "snake oil." We need to get our message out effectively and often.

- Develop and deliver with a positive twist the specific countermessages that address "the government," rationing, choice, affordability, and "the unknown," including "what's it going to cost me," health care in other countries, and "socialized medicine." It needs to be stressed that the delivery system will remain predominantly private, as it is now.

- Develop a plan to get maximum media exposure through a variety of strategies that we can afford, and get the timing correct. The opposition has megabucks, knows how to use proper timing, and can afford to buy space on prime time TV, not just at 3 a.m. Again, use professional help, develop a series of themes that seem hopeful, experiment, change course if they don't seem to be working, and concentrate efforts on those approaches that work.

- Prepare a series of position fliers that are brief, simple, easy to understand, and can be used to counter the misinformation and myths from the opposition. Give these materials wide circulation and try to be sure they are used in a timely manner, when an issue has the spotlight.

- Take advantage of every opportunity to rebut regressive proposals from the medical-industrial establishment—and in a timely manner: call-in radio, op-eds, letters to the editor, input at forums, a coordinated information bulletin board with alerts to activists and a method to stimulate specific action at the right moment so that it gets the most media exposure. We have the means for communication: the Internet. But we need some group or groups to coordinate the effort, to act as "command headquarters."

- Have a "quick-response" team, linked by the Internet, that can respond quickly to opportunities to get the message out and counter the other side's actions.

- Seek foundation support to get our message out, to educate the public.

- Recruit some famous people to be visible and outspoken in support of the cause. Win Harry and Louise to our side, "the better way."

- Target politicians and community leaders at every level to hear our message. There are potentially millions of *ad hoc* lobbyists (activists and short-changed patients) whose passion can make more of an impression than the calculated retorts from paid lobbyists.

- Be sure our message gets out to all the groups and "summits" that are thinking about universal coverage. If we are excluded, find ways to be sure our message is heard—from carefully targeting key people with personally presented information to (if necessary) public demonstrations or even civil disobedience.[6]

- Work together so that we coordinate the battle and target our efforts to where they will be most effective. There may be disagreements on strategies among different activist groups, but we should all strive to agree on the ultimate goal.

- Develop a nationwide network of activists and community people who are willing to be (1) local leaders and (2) foot soldiers for the cause.

- Convince the opposition to join us (see Chapter 12). Target specific groups that could be recruited to be allies in the cause: small business, human rights groups, church groups, unions, big business, sympathetic professional societies (perhaps in that order). Have a coordinated campaign to do the recruitment, probably on a state-by-state level.

- Convince state legislators that Health Care for All can save their states money by providing a method to limit Medicaid expenditures.

- Continue to work on state-level efforts, such as initiatives and legislation, because they help bring attention to the cause, make the issue visible at the local level, and educate the public. They may even represent our "best chance" as a step to reach national health insurance—or an end in itself if America espouses a federalist (state-by-state) approach. We should continue to encourage out-of-state activists to help bolster a state's cause.

- Appeal to a sense of community. "We're all in this together." The same argument should be made for affordability. We pay more for the uninsured in the long run because they delay needed care, come in sicker, and require more expensive treatment that we all, as a society, wind up paying for.

What I've outlined above looks challenging. It looks like a political campaign. And it is. Flexibility and the ability to have a rapid response will be key elements to assure success. We cannot ignore grassroots support even if a top-down effort at universal coverage, like a ballot initiative or legislation, succeeds. Experience teaches us that we must have the grassroots with us because the corporate interests have managed to reverse some short-lived victories in the past.

What we're lacking is effective and coordinated leadership—and money. The vested interests have an abundance of cash, but we have the passion and a just cause. However, if we want to be effective, we will need to work together and pool our resources, both human and financial. Unlike the pharmaceutical or insurance industries, we can't drop a few million dollars at a moment's notice to create a "front" organization or finance a publicity campaign.

We need to be wary of the corporate "moles" who sponsor sweet-sounding "summits" that go nowhere. Separating out the corporate infiltrators, the rest of us activists need to collaborate despite philosophical disagreements because it's an uphill battle. America remains clueless. We argue over the meaning of incremental, sometimes trying to distinguish such terms as "incremental" and "sequential" from "piecemeal." But we can agree to disagree, and work together effectively, if we all keep our attention on the prize: comprehensive and affordable health care for everyone in America, as with national health insurance or an improved Medicare for All. The ultimate "interest" we are pursuing is the best interest of every patient—and that's all of us. And, after all (as discussed later in Chapter 18), Health Care for All is an "incremental" step in itself; what we're really after is Good Health for All. On the way there, however, it would sure be encouraging to hear a roar from the stadium: "Give me an H!"

Summary of Key Points

- The system is stacked against the grassroots activists and the American people, but time is on their side.

- An increasing number of groups are pressing for meaningful change through a variety of mechanisms, including ballot initiatives and legislative action.

- There has been a worrisome recent trend to shift the goal away from universal coverage to "reducing the number of the uninsured."

- It will be a challenge involving widespread community efforts to win Health Care for All.

Chapter 15

National Health Insurance or Medicare for All: A Reality in Our Lifetime?

There's an anecdote that relates what happened to a health care activist who toiled for many years for the cause of universal coverage. When she died, she went to heaven where she met God at the pearly gates. "God," she asked, "will there ever be universal coverage for health care in America?" God pondered the question for a minute and then replied, "Yes, indeed, but not in my lifetime."

AT THE BEGINNING OF the twenty-first century, there seems to be a sense of frustration or even hopelessness over the prospect of ever getting to universal coverage. Especially distant is the hope for a truly seamless system that would include *everybody*, such as an improved Medicare for All. Yet, I somehow cannot put out of my mind—perhaps I am paranoid—that this aura of impossibility has been created and kept alive by the vested interests of the medical-industrial complex, the merchants of misinformation and myth.

Speaking to a special Congressional hearing, Marcia Angell, the former editor-in-chief of the *New England Journal of Medicine*, strongly decried as a myth the idea that America could not reach universal coverage using a single-payer system (see Chapter 1, Myth #13). Of course, there is a whole litany of myths about American health care (again, see Chapter 1), including, "We can get to universal coverage through an incremental approach."

The increased interest in universal coverage that began to be evident in the late '90s was expressed in a September 6, 1999, *New York Times* editorial. It called attention to ". . . this country's grievous failure to provide coverage for nearly one-sixth of its population . . . . The problem remains a vivid and embarrassing rebuke to American democracy." A later editorial from the same newspaper, published September 24, 2000, queried, ". . . If this moment—a moment of unprecedented economic prosperity and looming budget surpluses—is the wrong one for an aggressive move towards universal health insurance, when will it be right?" Although the projected budget surpluses are now ancient history, the need for universal coverage has not gone away. It's possible that the switch to "looming budget deficits" could inspire and accomplish what the surpluses could not.

It's Become Fashionable to Talk About Universal Coverage

SINCE THE LATE '90s—perhaps enough time had passed since the Clinton health plan collapsed—there has been a flurry of proposals to cover the uninsured. Many medical societies have come up with plans, as have foundations and institutes, such as the Commonwealth Fund and the Economic and Social Research Institute.[1] And a variety of "summits" have been convened to talk about the issue.

However, the gist of most of the new proposals has not really been "universal," despite the rhetoric. Simple, comprehensive, and understandable proposals, such as the 2001 call for "Medicare for All" from the Economic Policy Institute,[2] have been in the minority. There even seems to be a more recent trend to replace the term "universal coverage" with "reducing the number of uninsured." Such is the case with the $10 million advertising campaign initiated in February 2002 by a new coalition of 13 organizations called "Covering the Uninsured."[3] Single-payer, "one risk pool," and Medicare for All advocates seem to have been purposefully excluded, even uninvited, from national "summits" on universal coverage. Nancy Dickey, the former president of the American Medical Association (AMA), while speaking at a meeting of the American Public Health Association, seemed to indicate there wasn't even a place at the table for single-payer advocates.

My untrusting side makes me wonder if the chief sponsors of the "summits" on universal coverage—the AMA and the pharmaceutical industry—may have had a hidden agenda in mind when they excluded single-payer advocates from their deliberations. After all, the AMA has been steadfastly against solutions like an improved Medicare for All. Their official, and oft repeated, position is that, "Single-payer systems are not in the best interests of the public, physicians or the health care of this nation and should be strenuously resisted." The AMA has managed to derail every universal coverage proposal over the past nine decades. Somehow, despite their strong opposition, Medicare, the limited single-payer plan for Americans 65 years old and over, got through in 1965.

As for the pharmaceutical industry, a national health insurance plan could be a disaster for their bottom line—or so they think, though it might not be so bad for them. It could mean an end to their ability to exploit the market so as to assure the highest price for their products. Why should the vested interests support real change when they can do piecemeal approaches that basically keep the status quo? Minor modifications that only tweak the system allow them to keep their primacy in the market and their profits. To give the appearance of being good guys, they can talk about universal coverage and then dismiss it as being unrealistic.

So these powers that be (aka "the Evil Empire" of the health care industry) have created the myth that America cannot, and will not, accept Medicare for All, or the equivalent. Who controls the media? Who has the ear of politicians? Who has the money to drop a few million dollars on an advertising campaign to derail an effort at universal coverage or to sink a proposal to put meaningful pharmaceutical benefits into Medicare?

Even the executive director at my community health center, though an advocate for universal coverage, frequently expresses his skepticism. "Do you really think we'll have universal coverage anytime soon? In our lifetimes?" he asks. And a well-meaning caller to the Eugene, OR, NPR affiliate, where I participated in a talk show, asked about a compromise quasi-universal proposal, insuring all kids progressively from birth, while making the assumption that a quicker process to cover everyone was politically impossible.

Some of the proposals for so-called "universal coverage," such as the Commonwealth Fund's idea, which falls short of really being universal, remind me of what happened when the last great debate on universal coverage took place in 1993–94. Great minds in Washington argued over whether 95 percent or 92 percent coverage satisfied the criterion for universal. I'm convinced that if we adopt something like the Commonwealth Fund's proposal, we will only perpetuate the wastefulness and administrative complexity of the current system. And we will continue to exclude many of the patients whom I (and others who take care of the uninsured) see personally. Those are the people who fall between the cracks because of their incomes and/or eligibility criteria.

It reminds me of a young man in Oregon who related how he earned just a few dollars too much to qualify for the Oregon Health Plan, or the single mom from Eugene who was careful not to earn too much money so her children could continue to qualify for Medicaid. Including everybody automatically would be so simple, so fair, and save so much on administrative costs, that one would think it would be a no-brainer. But such inclusiveness would limit how the vested interests could game the system. Those interests, the very same interests that a Commonwealth Fund-type proposal would serve, would prefer to shift all high-risk patients to government-paid programs. The private sector would retain the low-risk people (the well)—the profitable segment of our population.

Why Don't the People Who Know Better Do Something?

WHAT IS MOST DISAPPOINTING to me is the lack of support—or is it resignation?—from people who deal on a daily basis with the uninsured. There is a wide gap between the rhetoric and action.

The U.S. Public Health Service (PHS) and the Health Resources Service Administration (HRSA) have a prominent campaign to reduce health disparities to zero. A major goal of the PHS' effort called *Healthy People 2010* is that all Americans will have health insurance coverage by that date (it was also an objective for *Healthy People 2000*). Since having health insurance would without doubt be the single most effective measure to reduce racial disparities in health care and improve health status, why do we see so little action from the people in community health centers and the PHS community in support of a solution like national health insurance?

They can't possibly fail to appreciate the lower rates of insurance coverage in minority groups. The Census Bureau figures for 1999 show uninsurance rates of 33.5 percent for Hispanics and 22 percent for blacks, compared to 11 percent for non-Hispanic whites. Sadly, these percentages have changed very little since this book's first publication, and the following statement still holds true. In March 2002, the Commonwealth Fund released a study assessing health care quality and minority Americans.[4] Their conclusion: "Perhaps most fundamental to ensuring quality medical care for minority Americans is the availability of affordable, comprehensive health insurance."

Are HRSA and the PHS, not to mention the National Association of Community Health Centers (NACHC), afraid to speak up because they are (to a greater or lesser degree) dependent upon an administration that does not officially support such a solution? Are they playing politics so they can be assured that they will continue to have their portion of the health care pie in our fragmented system? Or are they simply too tied up in their daily work, with endless hours spent in pursuit of grants? They chase grants to support one part of the puzzle, while they're trying to nail down a sub-program to tie together with some other program (both of which will expire in a year or two). All of these efforts are directed toward meeting the needs of their uninsured or inadequately insured patients. It would be great if all these efforts could go to benefit the patients in need instead of seeking ways to get through wasteful and often counterproductive administrative mazes.

There is also a general assumption, perhaps reinforced by the stand of the AMA, that physicians in general are opposed to the single-payer-type solution. But a national study of academic physicians, residents, and medical students published in the *New England Journal of Medicine* in 1999 revealed that 57 percent of the respondents felt the single-payer option "would offer the best care to the greatest number of people."[5] A 2001 survey of Massachusetts physicians (in a state where a 2000 ballot initiative for universal coverage lost by only a 4 percent margin) revealed that 66 percent of the physicians felt single payer was the preferred option for reform. However, only 51 percent thought that most physicians they knew supported it.

The Naysayers' Logic

OPPOSITION TO A TYPE of solution like national health insurance or an improved "Medicare for All" comes from people who object to giving government such a large role. They fail to realize that government is already footing the lion's share of our spending for health care. If we factor in the costs of Medicare, Medicaid, the Veterans Administration, the National Institutes of Health, the Defense Department, public hospitals, health departments, community and rural health centers, the tax subsidy to employer-supplied health insurance, the spending of state and local governments on premiums, and workmen's compensation, "government" spending already accounts for more than 60 percent of all health care spending in the United States.[6] Private employers contribute less than 20 percent to the overall costs, with individual spending making up the rest.

The naysayers say they don't like making health care "an entitlement" or a right. We as a nation, supposedly being more attuned to individualism, have not yet embraced the concept of health care as a human right—as has every other industrialized democracy. The detractors of national health insurance or "Medicare for All" prefer giving more prominence to the concept of "personal responsibility." Perhaps for them, responsibly paying your taxes, which pay for Medicare, doesn't count. However, it seems it's the rich folks and corporate America, like Enron, that are best at finding ways to avoid paying taxes.

Analyzed properly, the "personal responsibility" gig is an excuse to "blame the victims." A person who has paid his/her taxes has in essence paid a premium for a health insurance plan called Medicare. The fiscal responsibility has been met. And this concept is applicable whether it's Medicare for people over 65 or Medicare for All. That leaves the "personal responsibility" mantra as a ploy to (1) justify co-pays or (2) punish the poor, who often can't afford the co-pays and thus delay care.

The objections to national health insurance or Medicare for All are partly philosophical but largely economic. Of course, it's ironic that the AMA should be so anti-Medicare. Although recent high-handed HCFA (now CMS) tactics have made the doctors angry, there was a time when Medicare made the doctors rich— despite the AMA's original opposition to the program.

How about looking at this issue from the point of view that *really* counts, the interests of the American people? What are the real worries that we should be concerned about if we were to have a solution like an "improved Medicare for All"? A "single risk pool" with all 280 million Americans in, and nobody out. From the patients' (as well as the providers') viewpoints, the concerns would be:

- The level of bureaucracy. The degree of regulation needs to be appropriate to assure accountability but not be over-powering. Vast simplification, including everybody-in eligibility and a well-understood (and comprehensive) benefit package, should facilitate the process of design-ing a user-friendly system that minimizes bureaucracy. A system that is more transparent will also lessen the need for bureaucracy. And there must be built-in mechanisms to allow easy public input into the system. The type of bureaucracy embodied in today's Medicare is not accept-able and will require improvement.

- Flexibility. Build into the design a degree of local control and administration so that individual needs can be appro-priately addressed. The system design must include an ability to be responsive to changing needs, including ways to encourage and enhance research, training, and excellence in health care.

- The winds of politics. As with the current situation, politics can affect the whole system—especially financing. That's why the system should have a separate trust fund, insulated from being raided to serve other needs.

- Choice and access. Likely not real worries. Choice should be much improved, since a patient could have full choice of any provider, unlike the current system. As for access, it would also be greatly improved overall, although there could be some local variations in access when the financing mechanism changes.

- Inefficiency and corruption/fraud. These are the standard conservative's worries about anything that is "government-run." Health care in America is already so inefficient (with Medicare being perhaps the most financially efficient, even in its current state, see Chapter 1, Myth #4) that this aspect could only be made better with national health insurance or an improved Medicare for All. As for fraud, a transparent system with fewer complexities can only serve to diminish fraud (see Chapter 2). And as to the fear about being "government-run," the delivery system would remain predominantly private, as it is today.

- "Rationing" of services. A fear that with budget shortfalls there could be a compromise in the benefit package. Decisions on benefits belong in a public forum, and a mechanism to provide public input into the decision-making process must be built into any reforms.

The myth of "Why we can't have national health insurance, or Medicare for All," builds upon many other myths about America's health care system. The politically based and economically motivated rhetoric has been designed to subvert any real change. "Americans want more choice, Medicare is going broke, we don't want big government, we don't want more taxes." And even a call for "compassion" (versus justice). Plant doubt. Play on people's fears.

Is it possible, in the spirit of American free enterprise exemplified by Enron, HCA/Columbia, WorldCom, and the pharmaceutical giants who pay off smaller companies *not* to produce generics, that the major economic powers within the health industry got together and decided to systematically exclude solutions like national health insurance? Savvy as they are on health care, it's hard to believe that the economic powers of our health care industry do not realize, deep in their hearts, that a single-payer type of universal coverage, with "one risk pool," is what America needs. A parallel situation might be that of the tobacco industry, which for years denied that smoking caused cancer—even though they knew all along that it did. Like the tobacco industry, the health care industry knows that it is to its own economic interests to milk the system for as long as it can. And that's why a person like Tom Scully, the former administrator of CMS, could assert with a straight face, at a National Health Policy Conference in 2002, that even doing limited fixes to Medicare and Medicaid will take 10 to 25 years.

After all, our current health care system isn't wasteful to the insurance industry, the pharmaceutical companies, the for-profit HMOs and hospitals, and some of the more lucrative parts of the medical profession. They can maintain the standard litany of myths while they continue to oppose meaningful reforms, such as national health insurance or a real pharmaceutical benefit within Medicare. It may take a cataclysmic event, or maybe a combination of really adverse economic conditions as Joel Miller describes in his essay "The Perfect Storm"[7] to shake us up. Maybe then we'll see Health Care for All or even a single-payer type solution like national health insurance.

Summary of Key Points

- There may be a conspiracy of the "vested interests" to keep single-payer national health insurance off the table.

- An improved and expanded Medicare for All offers a good starting framework and/or conceptual model for an American system of universal coverage.

- Without affordable, comprehensive health insurance for everyone, the goal of "zero disparities" for minority health care will not be realized.

- "Government" already finances about 60 percent of all health care costs in the United States. Private employers contribute less than 20 percent.

- A litany of myths from the "vested interests" helps to block universal coverage and maintain the status quo.

- It may take a combination of cataclysmic events to act as a stimulus for real change.

Chapter 16

"Single Payer Will Not Fly": A Response[1]

"Single payer will not fly. Period. I favor it but it has no chance, none, nada, zero with Bush in and the Republicans in Congress. . . . My view is: forget about doing best. It is time to do better. Let's get something. Fifty years of waiting for a national health system has left tens of millions with nothing. . . . "

—Arthur Caplan, PhD, director of the Center for Bioethics at the University of Pennsylvania, October 2001, in an e-mail to Ida Hellander, MD, executive director of Physicians for a National Health Program

IS NATIONAL HEALTH INSURANCE, or "single-payer" reform a pipe dream in America? Should Americans be settling for something less? Often this "best" option, "best" at least from the viewpoint of the American people, is abruptly dismissed with a snicker and a curt "Forget it, it's politically impossible." I had to face that attitude recently when I was discussing a single-payer approach as one of the options for increasing coverage in Idaho. And I had to admit that—given the complexity of the whole issue and the level of understanding, as well as the philosophical bias of Idaho's politicians—it would be a hard sell. Idaho has the most Republican (89 percent) Legislature in America.

The myth that single payer is impossible in America has been propagated by special interests in order to cut off any discussion of single payer as an option (see Chapter 15). When a group of health care organizations put out their "Joint Statement" on universal coverage in 1999, they specifically specified that any solution had to be "pluralistic," thus automatically excluding the single-payer approach while mandating a "poison pill" that makes simplification of our fragmented system nearly impossible. Single-payer advocates were not even allowed at the discussion.

Does "Incremental" Have a Chance?

THE MYTH ASIDE, will a "something" solution cure our wasteful and badly fragmented health care system? Can we scrape together enough crumbs so that, even if we don't have the whole cake, the health care needs of the American people will be satisfied? I think these questions bring us back to the overall feasibility of "incremental" changes (see Chapter 1, Myth #12, for more discussion). Can "incremental" work? There's no doubt that incremental changes, though at best only marginally effective, are politically feasible. But our recent experiments with a series of incremental proposals have only seemed to buy time for the special interests, time during which the plight of the American people, and their access to health care, has only gotten worse. Some groups of Americans have been included (as with SCHIP, for example) while other groups (those millions with ever-increasing deductibles and co-pays) have been experiencing increased difficulty in accessing care.

We have experimented with (and continue to toy with) medical savings accounts (or health savings accounts), Medicare Advantage plans (formerly Medicare+Choice, which, ironically, has often meant less choice), Medicaid managed care, the SCHIP program, guaranteed issue insurance, small group insurance purchasing, catastrophic funds, and a variety of Medicaid expansions. The most current proposals *du jour* are now tax credits, "defined contributions," and high-deductible plans with health savings accounts. With the possible exception of the managed-care approaches, all of these incremental efforts have zero potential for changing a system that is broken. In fact, they fragment the system even more by making it even more complicated and administratively wasteful.

As for the managed-care approaches, such as Medicare Advantage plans, they have often only served to increase overall cost—the opposite of their intended goal. Moreover, they have led to an accentuation of the problem of risk avoidance, or "cherry picking," a problem that only a "single risk pool," or national health insurance, can solve. As for one of today's "poster child" solutions—refundable tax credits—the complexity of this proposal is so extreme that it is difficult to believe that serious thinkers can even realistically consider the option. Perhaps it would serve the interests of single-payer proponents to actually have a go at refundable tax credits. The resulting implosion of the financing system, which is headed toward meltdown anyway, would require a more radical fix, like national health insurance.

How About Affordability for the Patient?

INCREASINGLY, WE NEED TO deal with the question of affordability. And that question has two sides, one of which we have so far neglected to address as a nation. We have given attention to and worried about affordability from the viewpoint of our national and state budgets. And politicians have been sensitive to the increasing health insurance cost burden on business and industry. But in comparison to the attention given to costs for government and industry, almost no attention has been devoted to the cost of health care borne by the patient or consumer. Instead, the patient has been increasingly squeezed with a spiral of higher deductibles and co-payments. And people who have been sick are penalized even more, especially if they have an awful "pre-existing condition," with astronomical prices for health insurance, if it's even available. The "incremental" approaches have done nothing to improve this situation. Nor do such approaches have the potential to deal with these kinds of problems.

Admittedly, I am biased by the patients I see on a daily basis at my community health center—over half of whom are uninsured. When I consider my low-income patients, the various piecemeal proposals—health havings accounts, tax credits, and small group arrangements to buy bare-bones coverage—seem like pipe dreams as opposed to single payer. It totally depends on the angle from which one looks at what needs to be done. From the politicians' angle, influenced by the best information and biases that money can buy and a philosophy that holds on to the impossible dream that "the market" can solve our health care woes, single-payer national health insurance seems a political impossibility. Yet, to the American people (all of us who are patients/consumers, and especially those of us who are squeezed by health care costs or simply unable to afford health care at all), single-payer national health insurance is probably the *only* solution that will work. Other solutions, the incremental type, not only will continue to perpetuate an increasingly complex and wasteful system, but also will create new cracks in our already profusely leaking series of safety nets. If the American public really understood what the trade-offs were, they—instead of corporate America—could apply pressure to our politicians that would make national health insurance a political reality instead of a political pariah.

Consistent with our head-in-the-sand approach to international matters in general, we have ignored or purposively degraded through disinformation campaigns the experiences of other countries (Canada, for example). No foreign health care system is perfect, but the developed countries do cover everybody, and they do spend a fraction of what we spend—while we fail to cover more than 46 million Americans (an increase of over 6 million since 2000, with 3,200 people a day being added to the rolls) and expose even more to financial ruin should they be so unlucky as to incur a serious illness or injury.

The question remains, can we make the situation "better" without a "single risk pool" or without universal coverage? Even a state-by-state strategy or the expansion of Medicare to an entire age group, such as every child or everyone 55 to 64 years old, could serve as a starting point. But without a single-payer approach, we will just be playing the poke-the-balloon game, where pushing a finger in one spot just creates a blip on the other side.

"Best" vs. "Better": In Search of Value for Our Money

WE COULD ACCOMPLISH SOME changes, though I'm not sure it would meet the definition of "better," by throwing more money at the system. The simplest approach would be to increase eligibility for Medicaid or SCHIP, as many states have already done and as some national schemes propose (including the ACP-ASIM proposal for universal coverage), thus increasing the enrollment of low-income people in these plans. But Medicaid is very unpopular among politicians in most states and carries the stigma of "welfare." And states are now frantically trying to limit their Medicaid spending. Moreover, access to providers is limited because of its low reimbursement.

The fiscal implications would be significant, but if it's only a question of money, theoretically we could greatly expand Medicaid to cover, say, everyone up to 300 percent of the federal poverty level. Or we could simply buy commercial health insurance for every American, as the tax credit or rebate proposal tries to do, or as in Arthur Caplan's voucher proposal. That approach, however, wouldn't solve the problem for high-risk individuals or families, unless we were also willing to pick up their $1,000-a-month-with-$5,000-deductible premiums. The sky's the limit if we want to use our imagination and bankroll anything.

However, I think there's some political—and practical and ethical—advantage in getting some value for what we spend. And that value depends very much on having a cohesive financing system that can share the risk, set priorities, use scientific and information-based health care modalities (including prevention), and have some vision for what America needs. Our fragmented system does virtually none of the above. Nor does our system give a proper place to prevention (see the following chapter) in addressing the issue of affordability.

It appears likely that, at least for the immediate future, we will continue on the piecemeal track. Many, including myself, will work on proposals to make access "better," knowing that "better" is a slippery slope, perhaps leading nowhere. In time, possibly sooner rather than later, the stars will align to make the time right for national health insurance—likely *de facto* single payer but with some limited role for our insurance industry. The events of September 11 may have helped to bring into play some of the necessary change elements, such as a sense of community and some decrease in our disdain for government. But it will take a critical mass of hurting Americans—and a better public understanding of a complex issue—to create the grassroots groundswell that will make national health insurance politically acceptable.

Meanwhile, personally, I'll continue striving for "best"— national health insurance with "one risk pool"—because that's what my patients deserve.

Summary of Key Points

- Incremental changes can only be minimally effective in attaining meaningful health care reform.

- We will not have health care justice or affordability unless we include every person in America in "one risk pool," simplify the system, and reduce administrative costs—all impossible with the kinds of incremental approaches being proposed.

- Unless we choose the "best" solution—as opposed to piecemeal approaches—most of my patients will continue to do without needed health care.

Chapter 17

Needed for Affordable and Effective Health Care Reform in America: A Paradigm Shift for Prevention

The speaker at the closing day general session of the annual meeting of the American College of Preventive Medicine was expounding about how exercise as a routine way of life had not yet become mainstream in America. The day before, I had locked my bicycle to a bench across from the entrance to the five-star hotel in New Orleans where the meeting was being held. Hotel people snipped a cable lock and disassembled the bench so they could remove the bike, which they undoubtedly considered unworthy of gracing the front of their upscale hotel. When the speaker finished, I related—to the delight of the audience—the bike story to illustrate that America still has a long way to go to make exercise an accepted part of our daily lives. It's probably some consolation to remember that a mere 25 years ago, meetings of the College took place in smoke-filled rooms. Change can happen.

AFFORDABILITY IS A CRITICAL PART of the solution to making "Health Care for All" possible. And prevention—*real* prevention—has a key role (along with administrative savings) in making "Health Care for All" affordable. Although there is some controversy over how much some clinical preventive measures actually save overall, the more basic prevention activities, such as immunizations and prenatal care, have been clearly demonstrated to save money for our society as a whole. For example, it is generally agreed that for every dollar we spend on prenatal care, we save $7 in the long run. And a smoking cost study released in

229

April 2002 by the Centers for Disease Control and Prevention (CDC)[1] calculated how much money our society could save by reducing the use of tobacco products. The study put the nation's total cost of smoking at $157.7 billion a year, or $7 for every pack smoked, about evenly split between smoking-related medical costs and lost job productivity. Dealing with our nation's epidemic of obesity probably offers even greater possibilities for overall cost savings (see below).

The traditional medical care approach to assuring good health has its limits. New technologies have opened up a myriad of wonderful new possibilities for health care. And the future will undoubtedly see an increasing number of therapeutic advances capable of both improving and extending our lives—assuming we're fortunate enough to have access to them. But economic, environmental, societal, public health, and lifestyle changes have historically been the major factors in the betterment of our health status. And it's likely these nonmedical factors will continue to play a pivotal role in our nation's health in the future. Compared to the general public health efforts, many of the new medical/technological modalities tend to be much more expensive and narrower in their impact.

Prevention in the setting of overall community health, as opposed to clinical preventive medicine, which has its own more limited scope, is essential for the long-range success of any universal coverage plan. I'm not referring to "Putting Prevention Into Practice," the catchy phrase used to promote clinical preventive medicine. Rather, what I'm talking about is "Putting Prevention Into America." This more comprehensive brand of prevention deserves a much greater role in America's more global quest for "good health for all," as opposed to "health care for all."

America has experienced successes in prevention. Smoke-filled rooms are now a rarity in our society. There have been significant strides toward reducing the use of tobacco—despite some recent setbacks in cutting the rate of teen smoking. There has also been an increased awareness—accompanied by action—of the effects of environmental factors on our health. Decreases in deaths from motor vehicle accidents have come from preventive efforts in the form of safer highways and increased seat belt use. Improved housing as well as safe water and food have meant better health for Americans. By and large, these advances have been inspired by public health but have come through the political arena or as societal changes, and not through medical science.

However, as a society we have failed so far to come to grips with how we should deal with a host of chronic diseases like heart disease, strokes, obesity, arthritis, and diabetes. There is evidence that chronic diseases affect the uninsured much more adversely than people with coverage. A study by the Center for Studying Health System Change[2] found that the uninsured with chronic illnesses are three times more likely not to get the medical care they need. The May 3, 2006, *New England Journal of Medicine* and the July 2006 *American Journal of Public Health* revealed that compared to the British, Americans have higher rates of cancer, lung disease, and stroke with double the prevalence of diabetes and a 50 percent higher rate of heart disease. Compared to Americans, Canadians were 33 percent more likely to have a regular doctor and 27 percent less likely to have an unmet health need. Americans were also seven times more likely to report going without care because of cost. Meanwhile, there is a growing body of evidence that chronic diseases are preventable through lifestyle modifications. A prospective study published in February 2002[3] demonstrated that a program of moderate exercise and weight reduction led to a 58 percent decrease in the incidence of type 2 diabetes. Chronic diseases take a huge economic and human toll on the American people because so many millions of Americans suffer from them.

American society has evolved in a manner that has encouraged our current "epidemic" of chronic diseases. Part of the fault in our failure to deal effectively with chronic diseases through lifestyle changes (exercise, weight loss, quitting smoking, etc.) probably comes from having too much faith in medical science. Curative medicine has done wonders and is often capable of erasing many of our sins—at a price. If popping a pill can control your diabetes or clean the fat out of your arteries, why worry about being a couch potato? I had a patient who, after his quadruple cardiac bypass surgery, continued to smoke four packs of cigarettes a day and shun exercise. Why worry, when an artery can be reamed out with microsurgery? But medical science, which has provided antidotes for our own self-abuse, is only partially to blame.

As the speaker at the preventive medicine meeting stated, exercise has not yet become "mainstream" in America. In contrast, limiting the use of tobacco products has, as has the exposure to other environmental toxins. An article on transportation goals in Idaho's Treasure Valley (the area around Boise) appeared in *The Idaho Statesman* in December 2001. The "ambitious goal" in a 20-year plan for commuting was to get people out of their cars. For the "bike or walk" objective, the planners projected *no* growth—3 percent today, and for 20 years hence, still 3 percent. Reality? Maybe, but it's illustrative of the problem. As a society, we're clueless.

A Prime Example: America's Epidemic of Obesity

Anna is an 11-year-old Hispanic girl brought into the office by her mother with cramping abdominal pains and constipation. She is 4'8" and weighs 140 pounds. Her only physical activity occurs twice a week in her fifth grade physical education class. When at home, she watches "lots" of TV. Her diet includes "a lot" of candy and soda pop. A schoolmate, Marjorie, is 9 years old, in fourth grade, and weighs 177 pounds. Her only exercise is two sessions of P.E. a week; she consumes "munchies" and watches TV when she's at home. Her mother developed diabetes at a young age (35) and worries that Marjorie will too.

OUR GROWING EPIDEMIC OF OBESITY is a prime example of our society's failure to address the changing American diet and to make exercise "mainstream." Between 1991 and 2000, the prevalence of obesity in American adults increased by 61 percent—to 19.8 percent of all adults. The prevalence of morbid obesity—a body-mass index (BMI) of 40 or more—more than doubled in the same 9 years, from 0.9 percent to 2.1 percent.[4]

Internationally, we are winning first place in the contest for being the fattest nation. For the 24 OECD (Organisation for Economic Co-operation and Development) developed nations, the United States ranks number one—by far—in obesity for both men and women.[5]

Our society is paying a price for the huge increase in obesity, which also leads to more diabetes, heart disease, and worn-out joints. Now we're even seeing kids with type 2 diabetes, something we never saw 20 years ago. In December 2001, The U.S. Surgeon General came out with a report that attributed 300,000 deaths a year to obesity. He blamed most of the disaster on our increasingly sedentary lifestyle. Maybe people figure it doesn't really matter because they can always get insulin pumps, heart bypass grafts, organ transplants, or joint replacements. In the future, maybe people will be able to have beta-cell transplants (for diabetes), gene therapy, and mechanical hearts. But that line of thinking makes no logical (or economic) sense. Maybe, however, it helps to make us complacent. Something has happened to America to make us a sedentary nation. Why have we become so exercise-averse?

Paradoxically, we have seen an increase in the number of recreational centers in America—places where middle-class folks go to "work out." We seem to have spawned a subclass of exercise freaks who do workouts in gyms and run marathons. But the great bulk of Americans, notably those who have lower incomes or must work at more than one job to make ends meet, don't partake in the gym rituals. It's all part of the growing disparities in America, disparities based on economics that translate into heath status disparities.

There are many factors in American life, factors that have influenced our diet and our level of physical activity, that have accelerated our slide, as a nation, to "Fat City." Among them:

1. Literally, Fat City. The urbanization and/or suburbanization of American society.

2. Television and video games. Watching the football games instead of playing touch football, etc. With the exception of a growing elite (like the marathoners and triatheletes),

Americans are primarily "into" spectator sports. And while we watch, we eat.

3. Our dependence on the automobile—and our almost rabid protection of it as a way of life. I recall a letter to the editor while I was running for public office. Since it was widely known that I rode a bicycle, the writer attacked me, saying the "only way they'd get [him] to stop driving is when they peeled his dead hands off the steering wheel." With this kind of attitude as almost an axiom of American culture, we've seen barely more than token efforts to expand transportation systems based on human power. And we've built our communities in such a spread-out fashion as to make automobile use almost mandatory.

4. Lower wages for working-class people. There are fewer high-paying manufacturing jobs. More people are now working at lower-paying service jobs. Thus, they need to work longer and/or have several jobs. The result? No time or energy left to exercise. There's no time to walk somewhere. And time pressures necessitate using a car.

5. The decrease of physical education in the schools. Too many other demands. Meanwhile, kids in schools have easy access to candy and pop machines.6

6. The dominance of team sports (can lead to more joint replacements later) instead of lifetime sports.

7. Despite the increasing availability of "low-fat" foods, Americans, and especially low-income Americans, are taking in more calories. Low incomes and less time combine to increase the consumption of "fast foods." Compared to other countries, food—especially high-carbohydrate food— is cheap in America. One only needs to go to a buffet restaurant and observe plates piled 6 inches high with food to appreciate the American appetite. Even in non-buffet restaurants, the portion sizes have become humongous. We now have 44-ounce "Big Gulps" and "Colossal Burgers."

8. The commercialization of food, especially on TV. People are bombarded with TV ads selling a plethora of high-calorie snacks, drinks, etc. Food has become part of our American psyche—just as exercise has not.[7]

What Are the Side Effects of Making Exercise "Mainstream"?

IN ALL FAIRNESS TO AMERICA and Americans' attitude toward exercise, there has been some progress in how we look at exercise. The week after the people at the New Orleans hotel confiscated my bike (I got it back, of course), I rode it to another conference at a Marriott hotel in Portland, Oregon. I had biked 11 miles in a pouring rain, and my Gore-Tex suit was soaked. The hotel folks at the entryway invited me to put my bike and rain clothes in the valet's room next to the entrance to dry out. What a difference.

I suspect the exercise "gap" in America is part of the larger picture of health disparities, predominantly based on economic class and economic realities. But if we each took some positive action toward creating a society that really valued exercise, we could make real changes, much as we have with smoking and the environment. These changes do not have to take generations to work. They can be accomplished in decades if we have the will. For example, two simple strategies to lessen our dependence upon our automobiles would be: (1) increased investment in mass transit; and (2) making human-powered transportation safe, as with bike trails that connect so that commuting to work can be practical.

Unfortunately, the health care industry's "mainstream" players, with a few notable exceptions, are unlikely to profit from a paradigm shift in how America looks at exercise—or how we improve our diets. The pharmaceutical industry would be especially affected. With the growing epidemic of obesity, the drug companies can look forward to a financial windfall. Many millions of Americans will be taking their "statin" drugs to lower their cholesterol levels. And they could each be spending $3 a day, or $1,100 a year, for the rest of their lives. There are the similarly expensive "lifetime" drugs for diabetes, hypertension, and heart disease. People will be buying a wide variety of new look-alike but possibly safer (and more expensive) medications for pains in their stressed-out joints. The profit potential for safe new weight-reduction drugs is also phenomenal. And then there is the panoply of extraordinarily expensive medications, sometimes at several thousand dollars a dose, that accompany high-tech surgeries like the placement of cardiac stents or transplants. If I were a drug company CEO looking out for the financial welfare of my stockholders, I'd worry about exercise becoming "mainstream" in America. Ironically, the stockholders are probably the same people who can be found working out at the gyms.

I recently made an exercise-based suggestion to a sales "rep" from one of the large pharmaceutical corporations. He was at a diabetes meeting where he was marketing his company's drugs for diabetes and cholesterol. The latter has annual sales in the billions. I suggested that his company had a way to demonstrate just how much they really cared about the health of Americans. I proposed that his company donate a few billion dollars toward the promotion of community-oriented exercise in this country: media campaigns, funds for P.E. in schools, support for modifications in our transportation infrastructure to make human-powered commuting safe and practical. He thought it was a great idea. We actually will be working on it, but I won't be holding my breath until it happens.

Exercise as a national norm would likely also negatively affect the incomes of certain medical specialists, like cardiologists, cardiac surgeons, and endocrinologists. Orthopedists could probably break even, as sports injuries could take the place of what they earn replacing worn-out joints. At least their job would be more varied. Access to care would be easier, since doctors' offices wouldn't be so crowded with people who have diabetes, hypertension, obesity, and depression—the diagnoses that make up most of the practice of adult medicine. And hospitals and nursing homes would likely see census decreases as a result of a generally healthier population. Since exercise has a beneficial effect on mental health, especially depression, there would be less need to take care of depression medically, and there would be less demand on our inadequate mental health system. However, the drug companies would suffer. A year's treatment for depression with one drug typically costs about $1,000.

As for the insurance industry and the HMOs (assuming a status quo), they could come out ahead. They would pay out less money for procedures and medications because people would generally be healthier. With fewer "high-risk" people to avoid, they would be able to enroll more people in their plans. Prevention has traditionally received great "lip service" from the HMOs, but more often than not it has been used primarily as a marketing tool. They have used the clinical preventive medicine measures (immunization rates, for example) largely to sell their products. There has been little commitment (with some exceptions, as with Group Health of Puget Sound and their promotion of bicycle helmets) to change the way society looks at prevention in general.

Action Steps to "Put Prevention Into America"

WHAT HAS BEEN LACKING overall is real advocacy, in the form of personal commitment and financial support, for real prevention (exercise and diet modification being prime examples). Compared to the amount of money, the many billions of dollars, that go into the marketing of poor health habits by the "dark side" of American business, prevention gets a pittance. Even physicians, hassled by paperwork and tied up in their hectic daily routines, don't have the time or the foresight to "get involved" in actions that would really help their communities—and thereby their patients. But industry can find millions to sell Pepsi in schools or promote the "statin" drugs that lower cholesterol.

Real prevention could go a long way toward making America a much more humane society. What if we had a society with a higher degree of wellness? That could, of course, go along with a narrowing of the disparities between the well and the unwell in America, disparities that generally correlate with economic class. What if we had less stress in our society? Would our health indicators improve? What if we put more value on well-being than fancy homes, cars, and maximizing profits? Compare a one-and-

a-half-hour drive to work in stop-and-go traffic on an L.A. free-
way with a 10-minute bike ride to work in a small town in the
Midwest. Time spent talking on the phone in an office cubicle
versus time spent doing physical work in the outdoors. Or having
a modest dwelling and time to spend with family, as opposed to
not having the family time—or the time to exercise—because
long hours of work are required to meet high mortgage payments.

There are, of course, the direct positive health effects of exercise, and how these affect our overall humanity. We relate better
to each other if we're not depressed, not sick, not limping with a
worn-out knee joint, and more able to do our daily activities for
others and ourselves. Our physical and mental well-being is
directly related to physical activity. Yet exercise is still a "fringe"
activity for the majority of Americans. What can we do, as individuals and as a society, to make prevention "real" in America?
To cause a paradigm shift in how America looks at prevention,
and (more specifically) exercise?[8] Some practical action steps
include:

1. Convince American industry to invest in the promotion of
   prevention, especially to try to integrate exercise into the
   daily lives of Americans, including at the workplace. A
   practical example is the convenient placement of stairs—
   versus elevators.

2. Governmental support for the above, funded at no extra cost
   through cost-shifting away from sedentary transportation to
   human-powered transportation.

3. Urban planning that makes human-powered transportation
   practical and safe.

4. Increased physical education in schools, with an emphasis
   on lifetime physical activities, combined with a movement
   to have only healthy foods in schools.

5. Increased community-based efforts, with financial support
   from the private and public sectors, to promote physical
   activity for families, communities, and individuals.

6. Encouragement and participation of community leaders, including politicians and health professionals, in exercise-based activities that are not primarily competitive.

7. Increased public health outreach activities, especially in schools and in communities, to promote healthy lifestyles, especially physical activity and a healthy diet.

8. Appropriate taxation (or the opposite, positive financial incentives) to encourage healthy lifestyles, especially exercise as a routine activity. Examples: greatly increased tobacco, alcohol and gasoline taxes; taxing soft drinks; higher vehicle licensing fees. Conversely, subsidies and/or rewards for people who walk or bike to work, agricultural subsidies for the producers of fruits and vegetables—as opposed to the current subsidies for producers of tobacco and sugar.

9. A national campaign, looked at as "an investment in America," to promote prevention and exercise as goals that will improve our society's health and sense of well-being as well as make health care for everybody more affordable.

10. Research activities to document the effects of "Putting Prevention Into America" and making it truly mainstream.

As a matter of public policy, it makes unequivocal economic sense, for all the many reasons outlined above, to support efforts at all levels to make exercise "mainstream" in America. "Putting Prevention Into America," with the objective of making prevention, and especially physical activity, a new paradigm, will serve our nation well. Replacing the current paradigm that places a blind faith in medical science to "fix everything" would be a huge step forward. It would also be a key measure going "beyond universal coverage" to improve the health of Americans. It would make us a healthier and kinder society. And it would help make "Health Care for All" an affordable reality, not just a dream.

Summary of Key Points

- We have an epidemic of obesity in America, largely due to an increasingly sedentary lifestyle and poor eating habits.

- We are the "fattest" nation of all the developed countries.

- Unless we deal effectively with obesity and our lack of physical activity, we will see an ever-larger increase in chronic diseases such as diabetes, high blood pressure, heart problems, and strokes.

- We must strive to make physical activity "mainstream" in America.

- The long-term financial consequences of failing to deal with preventive measures will severely affect our ability to create an affordable health care system.

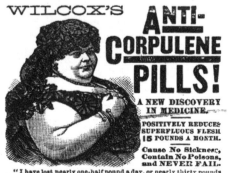

Chapter 18

Beyond Universal Coverage

Marian is the single mother of a teenager diagnosed with a bipolar disorder. Even though her employer provided health insurance, she was forced to leave a job of 11 years so that her son could receive Medicaid. She worried that her son might require extended hospitalization for his problem. If that happened, under her old insurance, which covered only a maximum of 8 days in the hospital, she would have had to pay the balance, probably tens of thousands of dollars out of pocket. At one point, her son's psychiatrist suggested that Marian turn over custody of her son to the state so he could be placed in a shelter home and thereby get Medicaid.

Marian had also been turned over to collection agencies by physicians who wouldn't accept payments. And she had to beg hospitals to write off parts of bills to avoid bankruptcy. When her son recently broke his jaw, her insurance would pay only 50 percent of the bill because the surgeon was not a "preferred provider." The insurance company failed to tell her that no pediatric surgeons in Idaho had agreed to be "preferred providers."

UNIVERSAL COVERAGE ALONE is not sufficient to reach the "desired outcome" of good health for everyone in America. But we can look at national health insurance or Health Care for All as a type of incremental change. A major step forward, but not a panacea for all that ails our health care system. It would be a boon for access to care. It would be undoubtedly the most essential step in decreasing health care disparities in America. But it wouldn't necessarily guarantee access, let alone good quality care. Look at Medicaid, for example. People with Medicaid—and Medicaid can have a very comprehensive benefit package—often have a difficult time finding physicians. Finding a dentist who will take Medicaid is more difficult yet. For those with Medicare, there is sometimes a problem with access, while minority Americans with Medicare have been shown to get less care.

Besides the lack of insurance coverage and/or financial barriers, there are other factors that affect the ability of Americans to get the health care they need. Those other obstacles include geographical access, cultural and linguistic barriers, shortages or maldistribution of certain kinds of health professionals (that is, nurses, dentists, and mental health workers), and even racism.[1] In addition, there are questions related to the scientific appropriateness of the care delivered. Transportation can be a major problem, as can a host of social circumstances that have an impact on health.

Community health centers like to think that they are "the specialists" in dealing with these "peripheral" but essential circumstances that affect the ability to get needed care. And, indeed, the health centers do represent more than just a "safety net" for the uninsured because of the "extra" services they provide. Even Canada, with its universal coverage, has community health centers to serve those "special" populations. Beyond coverage, to serve the health care needs of America, our system will need to address such issues as improving our information systems, increasing the practice of evidence-based medicine, eliminating medical errors, and taking more accountability for outcomes. We will also need to give increased attention to prevention—especially in the sweeping sense of societal change—without which we will continue to fall short in our pursuit of good health. We'll need to give a higher priority to such issues as pop machines and physical education in schools versus designing protocols for the use of cholesterol-lowering drugs. Deciding which people need their carotid arteries reamed out is important, but it makes much more sense to invest more of our resources in finding ways to provide kids with positive alternatives to watching TV and playing video games.

Assuring Adequate Coverage

U NIVERSAL COVERAGE MUST INCLUDE a comprehensive and adequate package of benefits that meets the health care needs of all Americans or it will be a "sham" endeavor. At the very least, it must cover inpatient and outpatient care, emergency care, mental health, diagnostic and lab tests, long-term care, basic dental and eye care, pharmaceuticals, adequate home health services, and necessary medical equipment.

At our evening clinic, I saw a middle-aged Mexican-American man who had brought in his daughter for an earache. As I finished giving him instructions on what to do for his daughter, he pulled out a sheaf of papers and asked if I could give an opinion. What he showed me was a health insurance policy for which he was paying $39 a month. Its main benefit was $50 a day for hospitalizations. Was this man insured? I wonder if he was one of the people polled by the Census Bureau when they calculated the number of uninsured Americans.

Then there is the issue of deductibles and co-pays, which has been addressed earlier (see Chapter 6)—the "personal responsibility" smokescreen. Of course, we should all exercise more, drink less, wear our seat belts, and not smoke at all. But all those obvious measures are not why the experts and the corporate types are pushing "personal responsibility." They're promoting it because they want a sweet-sounding excuse for shifting costs to the patient/employee. For less well-to-do patients, shifted costs often mean delaying or omitting care—even when it's necessary. It means a multitiered system, where the rich get one kind of care, the poor get another. Guess who would get the plan that has more comprehensive and timely care with fewer barriers?

There is an inconsistency in the call for outcome accountability and the use of scientific methods with the promotion of "personal responsibility" in the form of higher costs for patients. As mentioned above, I don't know of any scientific evidence showing that deductibles and co-pays produce better outcomes. Nor am I aware of studies proving that even higher deductibles and co-pays bring even better results.

Perhaps the health policy wonks, in their wisdom, have concluded that the use or overuse of services (whether necessary or not) is a risky affair. They may, not without some reason, fear that the very use of services will generate a certain degree of iatrogenic (self-caused) bad outcomes. But I don't think they have that much insight, and I do think it's all about money and short-term savings that accrue to employers and insurers, as opposed to patients or employees. Again, there is a lack of appreciation for the fact that delayed or omitted care costs more for everybody in the long run. The bottom line: any universal coverage plan must deal with the problem of deductibles and co-pays so that access to care for people with marginal incomes, as well as middle-class people, is not adversely affected. We will address this issue again in the Conclusion section of this book.

Reclaiming Dignity

THE NEW SYSTEM must allow people dignity. How people are treated and how they feel about themselves is important. A system of universal coverage with everyone in the same risk pool would eliminate the stigma that goes with Medicaid and the degree of disdain or rejection that some people with Medicaid (and the uninsured) must currently endure. Real universal coverage, as opposed to a stratified multitiered system that allowed the rich one kind of care and the poor another, would help return a sense of dignity to individuals. It's the same kind of dignity that Medicare provides for our elderly population. Only it would be better, since Medicare has evolved into an incomplete system. Universal coverage would help restore a sense of dignity to our nation. In the eyes of the rest of the world, America has become ethically "tainted" because of our failure to provide health insurance for everyone, as all the other developed countries do.

I was sitting next to a Canadian on a flight to Seattle a few years ago. We talked a bit about health care, and he said, "You know, I admire you Americans for many things, but, for the life of me, I can't understand why you don't have universal coverage." I've talked to Europeans who think we're barbaric because we actually allow someone to go bankrupt because he or she had the misfortune to be sick or injured. It amazes me that we've become so clueless to the fundamental issues surrounding health care that well-meaning Americans, who consider themselves to be caring beings, can sense nothing wrong about saying, "I think it's okay that Americans who can afford health care can get it, whereas those who aren't able to afford it can't."

Keeping America Clueless

THE MEDICAL-INDUSTRIAL COMPLEX has a financial stake in keeping America clueless about how our health system fails us as individuals and as a nation. As we have seen, the United States far exceeds our Western World neighbors in both per capita as well as percentage of gross domestic product health care spending. Yet we continue to rank in the twenties and thirties for most health indicators. We get poor value for all our spending. We Americans have been conned into believing that "we have the best health system in the world," along with a host of other myths (see Chapter 1). The mythology is not accidental. The spreading and maintenance of the myths has been bankrolled by the vested interests. The millions spent by the AMA in the early '90s to discredit Canada's system, the many more millions spent in 2000 by the pharmaceutical industry on "the bus from Canada," and the millions spent on "Harry and Louise" by the insurance industry and small business to kill Clinton's plan (bad as it was) are but a few examples of the concerted and directed effort to kill or delay meaningful health care reform.

These efforts to keep America clueless have been amazingly successful—to the point of having created inner (almost) dogmas that inhibit rational thought. This programmed mythology has implanted certain catchwords in our collective American psyche. In seemingly rational discussions about health care, throwing in phrases like "socialized medicine," "the federal government," "rationing," "taxes," "Great Britain," or "Canada" brings discussion to a screeching halt. Minds close. Even "universal coverage" and "health care reform" have become equated with socialism, and Americans certainly don't want *that*.

The issue of health care in America has become so complex that a few million media dollars to plant doubt can block significant change. Part of the ease in derailing new ideas comes from the relative lack of involvement of Americans in health care as an issue. Unless someone is ill or injured, there is little interaction with the system or appreciation for how it *doesn't* work.

The degree of cluelessness is amazing. It envelops our citizenry, much of the media, health care professionals, politicians, and the health care industry in general. It even touches many of the health policy gurus, who, in their academic world of ecnomic theory, often have little sense of what it means to lose your dignity in a dysfunctional health care system. Only after they've been sick and had the misfortune to experience the crazy side of American health care, as did Paul Ellwood (one of the original chief gurus of managed care), do they wake up and realize something has gone wrong. Many thinking people, including consultants and people from the insurance industry who have worked in health care for decades, appreciate the need for meaningful reform with "one risk pool." Most of them are of the mind that we need to go through more pain (more futile incremental or piecemeal approaches) before there will be a more general recognition of the need for truly universal coverage with one risk pool.

Although the events of 9/11 reminded us of our potential to share some values as a community, it will take a stronger sense of "community responsibility" (as opposed to "personal responsibility") to assure that every person in America has access to health care. Even in the face of strong economic arguments for universal coverage—every study done shows it would save us money—there is reluctance to bite the bullet and move forward. Whenever the moneyed interests perceive a threat to their empires, they spring to action to befuddle us and keep us clueless—as they tried to do with the November 2001 Portland, Maine, referendum for single-payer health care reform. The vested interests lost that referendum, but they'll be back to protect their "bottom lines" and keep us clueless.

The Global Picture

THE AMERICAN QUANDARY WITH Health Care for All, as well as the looming "meltdown" of our health care system, is really only a part of the larger picture. At the beginning of the twenty-first century, a worldwide struggle is taking place over the role of "globalization." In polarizing terms, the conflict could be described as one between the multinational corporations and the working people of the world. Of course, that's too simple a definition. But it does come down to a battle between the "haves" and the "have-nots," with the "haves" telling the "have-nots" they should have faith in free markets, capitalism, privatization, free trade, etc. Around the world, the efforts of the International Monetary Fund—notably their "structural readjustment" or privatization plans—have had disastrous results for working people. The rich have gotten richer, and the poor poorer. A recent example of the effects of privatization gone awry is the economic collapse in Argentina. Ironically, Argentina used to have a respected and responsive publicly administered health care system. Much of that system has now been privatized, resulting in markedly decreased access to health care for most Argentines.

What's happening in America's health care system today is, of course, influenced by the kind of thinking that has occurred with the world's shift towards globalization. The value conflicts are similar. The private versus public arguments. Health care as a right versus "the market."

Health care cannot really be viewed in a vacuum. It interrelates with other social and economic issues, such as poverty, hunger, racism, a living wage, adequate housing, and education. In a larger context, our current dilemma with health care raises the whole issue of whether, as a community, we have some responsibility to care for each other—as opposed to "personal responsibility." This "community responsibility" question applies to all the other problem social issues as well. On a perhaps more radical bent, some, including author Barbara Ehrenreich, have asserted, "The 'working poor' . . . are in fact the major philanthropists of our society. They neglect their own children so the children of others will be cared for. . . ."[2] The inequities and disparities in health care are perhaps the most egregious shortcoming of American society today because of the huge impact they have on so many millions of people.

Unless there is some reversal of direction soon, America's health care seems to be headed increasingly towards greater discrepancies between rich and poor as we progressively become a "culture of extreme inequality."[3] We seem to be lacking leadership as we drift towards a multitiered health care system. A system where the very rich will receive "concierge care," while the poor could be relegated to a phone card that will give them an hour a month of consultation with a "Dial-a-Nurse" service in Minneapolis or Bangalore.

Steps We Must Take as a Responsible Nation to Improve the Health of Our Communities

IF WE ARE TO MOVE FORWARD, "right the wrong," make health care affordable and accessible for every person in America, improve the health of our nation, and remedy the loss of dignity that we have inflicted on ourselves as individuals and as a nation, there are some specific actions we need to take.

1. As the first step—and one without which the rest will be more difficult to implement—we must have universal coverage. Everybody in, nobody out.

2. That universal coverage needs to be based on a "single risk pool" or it will *de facto* not be truly universal, as it will be gamed to exclude people who are high risk. Without the "single risk pool" there will be a multitiered system with its inherent inequities.

3. We need a paradigm shift in how we deal with health care and health. A change from the curative to the preventive. We currently overfund the curative and seriously underfund the preventive—perhaps by a ratio of 100:1. "Preventive" must include not just clinical preventive measures, but also strive for more comprehensive societal change (with the adequate allocation of resources). It's not just "putting prevention into practice." It's putting prevention into life.

4. Part of that prevention is minimizing delayed care and health care disparities. The key measure to reach these goals is universal coverage, but there are other barriers that must be addressed as well (see above).

5. Health care needs to return to an emphasis on health, not cost or profit. It should be regarded as a "public good," not a commodity. The pursuit of profit through health care produces twisted incentives that only lead to poorer outcomes, injustice, and discrimination. The goal should be health, not wealth. In the process, we need to assure that the quality of that health care is good and that our nation receives good value for what we spend on health care.

6. There should be grassroots efforts to define community priorities, assure community involvement and action, and inform the clueless. The American people should understand who the "modern-day snake oil merchants" are and what motivates them.

7. Harry and Louise should be recruited away from the "Dark Side" of health care and be used nationwide to combat the merchants of misinformation and myth.

8. Instead of using the mantra of "personal responsibility" to blame the victims, we should place a much higher value on "community responsibility" and restoring personal dignity. We also need to assure "corporate responsibility" in health care—or have them convert to a not-for-profit status—an idea that needs to be explored seriously.

9. The system needs to be simplified, not made more complex. Complexity is a barrier in itself.

10. As a nation, we need to recognize that national health insurance or Health Care for All is good for the American economy, perhaps the only way to avoid the meltdown of our health care system, and (most important) the "right thing to do." Health Care for All will help not only individuals, but also our nation, regain the dignity we have lost because of our health care system's egregious inequities and shortcomings.

Summary of Key Points

- Universal coverage (or Health Care for All) is only the first step toward a larger goal: good health for all.

- The benefit package must be comprehensive and adequate enough to address the real health care needs of all Americans.

- We must educate all Americans about health and health care to counter the efforts of the medical-industrial complex to "keep America clueless."

- We need to give more importance to "community responsibility" as opposed to "personal responsibility."

- Health care should be regarded as a "public good," not a commodity.

- There are many other factors that we will need to address in order to assure good health for everyone—including poverty, racism, education, decent housing, a living wage, the scientific basis of medicine, and effective prevention.

- Without Health Care for All, we will not regain our dignity as a nation.

The Fox and the Henhouse
by C. Rocky White

As one can see after reading Chapter 7, I do feel strongly about the humanitarian aspects of health care reform but, honestly, I did not arrive at my opinion on the need for a single-payer system through lofty ideals of social justice. Instead, it is a result of an understanding of sound medical business principles and years of working within a system infested with waste, inefficiency, and a broad maldistribution of resources.

The art and the practice of alleviating human suffering is at least as old as civilization itself. But the ability to incorporate sound medical science into a profession that could actually do something concrete to treat disease and prolong life is a relatively recent phenomenon. And, up until recent Western history, it was physicians who controlled the practice of medicine. Hospitals and asylums were predominantly a charitable outreach and extension of the church.[1]

For good or ill, the ability to actually intervene effectively has come with a price tag. For every advancement in medical science, the cost of health care advanced that much more. From the early twentieth century on, Western medicine began its evolution into big business, and clever entrepreneurs outside of medicine proper began to see the potential for profit.

The health insurance industry was one such extension, albeit at that time in history a necessary one. In fact, in the days when doctors could do little more than hold your hand and "humor the patient," workers could purchase sickness insurance, which would cover lost wages as a result of illness and funeral expenses when the physician's humor had expired.

As the cost of health care rose, insuring against expensive medical bills became a natural growth industry. During World War II, as wage freezes were set into place, manufacturing industries offered health care benefits as a way to lure workers. When our soldiers came home and the U.S. economy began its resurgence, the strategy to offer health care benefits to recruit and retain good employees became entrenched in corporate offerings and labor union expectations. Employer-sponsored health insurance became an expected part of any benefits package and the mainstay of coverage for most Americans.

However, the discussions about a National Health Program were never far away from the platform issues of mainstream politics. Nearly every decade of the twentieth century either had a president (from Theodore Roosevelt all the way to Bill Clinton) or a Congress that was willing to discuss or even pass bills out of committee and onto the floor of the Legislature in an attempt to create a national universal health care program.

This political discussion finally culminated in a compromise in the mid-1960s when Medicaid (coverage for the poor) and Medicare (coverage for the elderly) were implemented. These were the two groups felt to be the most vulnerable in terms of health care coverage, as they were the population entities most likely to not be covered by employer-sponsored insurance. In fact, any meaningful national debate on a universal health care system faded from the scene after 1965 and would not reappear with serious debate until the Clinton administration in the 1990s.

Maintaining health insurance in the private sector was felt to be more in line with the American values of freedom from government interference and the preservation of a free market. Also, any policy issue that rose for debate in the mid-twentieth century that strove to cover every American fell prey to anti-communist rhetoric and the fear that "socialized medicine" would be the next logical progression in surrender to the Soviet Union.

As the decades leading to the new millennium passed, the capital needed to fuel the medical industry increased, and the potential for profits at the fringes of the system became more apparent. More and more, health insurance companies converted to "for-profit status," merged and grew, and finally morphed into the multi-billion-dollar corporate conglomerate industry that we have today.

Another prime example of ingenious entrepreneurs recognizing the excessive fat in our system first came to my attention several years ago when my wife, a marketer, was working with a health care marketing research group. One day, she asked the company's CEO why the health care field was chosen as their primary client base. A big smile ran across his face and he replied, "Because that's the field with the biggest squeeze!"

Now, the first question to ask is, "Is there anything wrong with that?" After all, this is America. Capitalism and a free market are what have made the United States what it is today. There is nothing wrong with making a profit. In fact, some of the most flaming, liberal old hippies I know watch their 401(k) plans like a hawk as they approach impending retirement.

But!

When the profits and market control of one industry begin to drain and impede the growth and sustainability of all other industries, and the health and well-being of our nation is being sacrificed for the sake of "preserving free enterprise," it is time to readjust our priorities. We as a nation have breached that threshold.

As I travel around the country speaking on the subject of a universal health care system, I always like to make three points perfectly clear:

1. There is no evil empire. Every player in the health care industry is contributing in one way or another to out-of-control costs, and they all must be reined in.

2. Every aspect of our present health care system is broken and in need of reform.

3. Universal health care also means universal reform—from the way government manages entitlements to the way doctors and hospitals deliver care, from malpractice to the management of medical infrastructure, and everything in between.

But, first and foremost, until the profit motive of health care financing is eliminated, all attempts to reform and create universal access to health care will be cost-prohibitive and will be in vain.

Because employer-sponsored health benefits and the insurance companies that supply them have been a part of our culture for so long, it would seem only natural that we should look to this segment of the economy to apply market pressure in our search for reform. Since Ronald Reagan began to reprioritize government spending in the 1980s, the prevailing attitude in Washington has been to limit government and privatize as much of the economy as possible. This policy, in part, helped to bring about one of the most dramatic periods of sustained economic growth in our history.

There are those who argue that government programs yield nothing but burgeoning bureaucracies that stifle innovation and that all we have to do is keep as many health care dollars as possible in the private sector and the markets will readjust themselves.

There is just one problem: health care doesn't follow Wall Street economics. If it did, we wouldn't be having this discussion, and you wouldn't be reading this book.

For doctors, hospitals, and the patients they serve, there is no free market (not if you truly provide quality care to all comers). And as such, there is no place to apply market pressure. Any attempt to do so does not control cost; it simply shifts it to another segment of the system.

Let's start with competition. As a businessman, I love competition. It is the fuel that drives innovation in business. In health care we also have competition; it is what I call competitive avoidance. It is a perverse inversion of how we understand the market system and is a result of a multitiered, fragmented method of financing. It forces doctors and hospitals to not compete with one another on quality, outcomes, or patient safety (which is what medicine is supposed to be about). Instead, they compete for demographics and to see who can most successfully avoid the poorest-paying patients.

Evidence of this is all around us. How many hospitals in your metro area have closed their emergency rooms (where the poor and uninsured usually end up for care) in the last 5 years? Have you noticed where the newest hospitals and doctors' offices are being built? Is it in the parts of town where people are more apt to have good health insurance and are able to pay their deductibles?

And what about those "specialty hospitals" that cater only to orthopedics or cardiology, which coincidentally have some of the highest-paying procedures in the industry? They claim that if they focus on only one specialty, they can provide the highest quality care for the best price. The reality is that they can corner the market on the best-paying procedures and limit their exposure to patients who are at the highest risk for expensive complications. Also, they can avoid taking care of the poorly insured by not opening themselves up to admitting these patients through a well-advertised emergency room. These types of patients are shifted over to general hospitals, which are typically not-for-profit.

The same thing happens in outpatient clinics as well. As the metro sprawl moves continually outward, it leaves behind large pockets of the working poor and elderly. Physicians who are able to follow the sprawl into communities of well-insured and affluent families can then effectively build "fire walls" around their practices to keep out the poorly insured.

Now, I cannot blame the doctors. After all, they are just trying to survive in this perverted and convoluted system that we have created. But what ends up happening is that low-risk, well-insured patients end up pooling into small pockets, and everyone else is shifted over to government programs, community health centers, and not-for-profit community hospitals that are constantly struggling for funding.

In remote rural areas, the story is not much different, except that doctors and hospitals cannot "follow the sprawl" or build fire walls. They are just stuck with the patient population that they have. In the case of my clinic, the payer mix was so unfavorable that we could no longer afford to keep our doors open—we went broke providing quality health care and, incidentally, we had no one to compete against!

This phenomenon of inverted competition reminds me of the story of two buddies who went fly fishing on Alaska's Yukon River. After a morning of hard fishing, they waded up on a sand-bar to eat lunch. As they sat down and started to rummage through their packs, one of them noticed his buddy was taking out a pair of tennis shoes.

"Hey," he said. "What on earth are you doing with a pair of tennis shoes clear out here?"

"Oh, these? They're just in case we come across a hungry grizzly bear."

"Get real," the first one replied. "You don't hon-estly think that you can outrun a hungry grizzly!"

"Nope," the second shot back. "All I have to do is outrun you!"

Sadly, this perverse system of competitive avoidance is the same philosophy that drives the markets of the health insurance industry. They are only interested in recruiting low-risk, young, healthy patients and doing everything in their power to shift older, chronically ill patients out of their coverage and over to government programs or into the folds of the uninsured.

This perpetual game of hot potato is one of the main reasons (although not the only one) why placing the financing of health care in the hands of private industry cannot and will not allow the market to adjust itself.

Everyone in the industry, conservatives and liberals alike, recognizes the need for reform. Over the past few years, policy wonks from both ends of the spectrum have been number crunching in an attempt to find a workable solution. Although this country still has no consensus on an answer, there are several general points that are agreed upon by all:

1. The present system is irrevocably broken.

2. The system needs to be overhauled.

3. The system is eroding the economic fabric of the working class.

4. The system is impeding the effective competitiveness of business.

5. Nearly every American is being negatively affected and wants the system fixed.

6. There is only a finite amount of resources available for health care.

Because most are beginning to realize that the first step toward any type of cost containment requires that everyone have some type of insurance, the term "universal coverage" has now entered the vernacular of nearly every constituency looking at reform—including the insurance industry.

As a result, the options for reform requiring universal coverage are settling into two main philosophical camps:

1. A system that is publicly financed and accountable to the people.

2. Universal coverage through a multitiered, fragmented system, financed through a combination of private and public funding (which at this point represents the path of least resistance and supposedly is the most politically feasible).

Enter America's Health Insurance Plans (AHIP). AHIP is the single most powerful political voice of the health insurance industry and is one of the most respected and influential lobbies in Washington, D. C. It ranks a close second, if not equal, to the political influence of the American Medical Association (AMA). Suffice it to say that if AHIP and the AMA come together on a policy issue, any politician would be hard pressed to run askew of their combined lobby, no matter what the views of the general public may be.

I know firsthand what these groups are able to accomplish. As a physician and a medical director of an HMO, I have been a member of both. They are not bad organizations; in fact, they have accomplished a lot of good over the years. But their tenacious and single-minded lobby to follow the policy of for-profit financing of health care is going to drive this system into ruination. As the old man used to say, "Even the old cowboy had enough sense to know that when you find yourself in a hole, the first thing you do is stop digging!"

In November 2006, AHIP released a policy statement entitled "We Believe." It is an outline for a universal coverage plan and how it can be implemented at both a state and federal level over the next 10 years. The reason I have chosen this plan for the remainder of our discussion is that, at present, this appears to represent the most politically feasible idea and is the vanguard plan for anyone trying to avoid the discussion of a single-payer system.

The AHIP plan is, for the most part, very similar to what we all now know as the Massachusetts plan. It is also similar to what was introduced by Senator John Kerry in a speech he gave at Faneuil Hall in July 2006, and it seems to be the prevailing idea being carried by many politicians who are jockeying for the next election cycle.

Since these ideas seem to be the direction that political feasibility is heading, let's examine the AHIP plan in detail, remove the veneer of glossy rhetoric, and see if these concepts truly are a workable plan for reform.

"We Believe: A Vision for Reform"[2]

"The AHIP proposal is built upon 5 principles to be implemented in 3 stages with a time line of 10 years to phase it in.

Phase 1 (Years 1-3)
- Achieve coverage of substantially all children in each state.
- Achieve a 33 percent reduction in the number of uninsured adults.

Phase 2 (Years 4-6)
- Achieve a 66 percent reduction in the number of uninsured adults.
- Begin the process of extending Medicaid eligibility to all adults with incomes less than 100 percent of the Federal Poverty Level (FPL).

Phase 3 (Years 7-10)
- Cover all adults with incomes less than 100 percent of the FPL under the Medicaid program.
- Achieve coverage of at least 95 percent of adults.

Principle 1: The federal government should provide incentives to states to develop strategies that lead to—and sustain—coverage of children within three years and adults within 10 years.

Principle 2: The federal government should establish incentives for states to provide coverage through the Medicaid program for all adults with incomes under 100 percent of the federal poverty level (FPL), including single adults, and through the State Children's Health Insurance Program (SCHIP) for children under 200 percent of the FPL. States should have the option to exceed these levels for SCHIP to the extent necessary to maintain enrollment of existing populations.

Principle 3: The federal government should provide subsidies for the purchase of private coverage to individuals and families with incomes under 400 percent of the FPL. Individuals with incomes under 300 percent of the FPL should receive proportionally greater assistance, with assistance levels phasing down for individuals with incomes approaching 400 percent of the FPL. Individuals who are eligible for premium subsidies should be encouraged to purchase coverage through existing market mechanisms. Employed individuals who are eligible for employer-sponsored coverage should be encouraged to use their premium subsidies to enroll in such coverage.

Principle 4: The 6 million uninsured Americans with incomes over 400 percent of the FPL should be encouraged to purchase coverage. This proposal sets out a range of options states should consider to achieve this goal. To help create a level playing field for individuals purchasing coverage on their own and for those who have employer coverage, full tax deductibility of premiums purchased in the individual market should be granted.

Principle 5: Employers should be encouraged to facilitate, provide, and maintain coverage for their employees. This proposal sets out a range of options states should consider to
achieve this goal. In addition, the federal government should
not disrupt employer coverage by changing the current tax
treatment of employer-provided coverage."

(For more information or to review the entire AHIP proposal, go
to www.ahipbelieves.com.)

Notice that the first three principles place emphasis on the
federal government ("the federal government should . . ."). By its
own admission, the AHIP spells out that it is the role of government, not AHIP, to provide the incentives for everyone to have
health care coverage. (I thought the argument against a single-
payer system was to minimize the role of government in the
financing of health care. This proposal actually expands it—dramatically.)

Remember, the health insurance industry is not in the business of providing quality, affordable health care. They are in the
business of making money. We soon will see how this proposal
intends to further amplify their profits.

The first three principles call for the government to greatly
expand the current entitlement programs of Medicaid and the
State Children's Health Insurance Program (SCHIP). In 2006,
these programs already have exceeded $180 billion in federal
spending with just about that same amount being matched by the
states.[3] It then calls for additional government monies so that
those individuals who sit between Medicaid-eligible and those
with incomes at or below 400 percent of the FPL will receive
money in the form of tax vouchers or subsidies to purchase insurance. Purchase insurance from whom? The insurance industry, of
course.

Principles 4 and 5 then lay out how the government should
provide incentives (the presumption here is mandatory purchasing of private insurance) for employer groups and those with
incomes greater than 400 percent of the FPL. It calls for the

establishment of a Universal Health Account (UHA) to which people can make contributions and then use those funds to go toward their co-pays and deductibles for the high-deductible plans they are mandated to purchase. Since most Americans are already disgusted with the concept of health savings accounts (HSAs), we just change the name and use the word "universal" and already we are feeling better. Now, however, the healthy and wealthy can use their UHA as a retirement tax shelter.

Now, granted the AHIP proposal does call for the government to establish a match for contributions to the UHA of 50 percent up to a maximum of $2,000 for families below 300 percent of the FPL and a 25 percent match for those between 300 to 400 percent of the FPL. Remember, these proposals represent a match.

Do you realize that 300 percent of the FPL for a family of four is only $58,000 a year? That may seem like a reasonable income, but the annual insurance premium for a family of four now averages more than $10,000 a year. Even if the government were to pay half of the family's premium in the form of a subsidy and a $2,000 match towards a UHA, that still amounts to $7,000 a year for which that family is responsible—an amount that exceeds 10 percent of that family's income. Economists tell us that any time a family exceeds 10 percent of its income on health care expenditures, it is placing itself in a very financially vulnerable position.[4, 5] If the family carries a plan that provides a $2,000 deductible per person per year and it can't afford the match, and if a family member breaks a leg, they're done. It will bankrupt the family. Furthermore, it is the doctors and the hospitals that will eat the losses. But the insurance company will still be raking in the profits—with your tax dollars.

Also, this does not take into account the huge tax increases that will be felt by these working middle class families in order to fund this insurance industry pork barrel.

Through all of these proposals we keep seeing the words "tax subsidies," "expansion," and "incentives." Nowhere does the AHIP suggest where all this money is going to come from. But the beauty of this plan is that all those tax vouchers and subsidies are going straight into the pockets of the insurance industry for them to "manage." You don't need a PhD in economics to realize where it is all going to funnel to, with an industry average overhead and profit-taking of 20 percent.

The AHIP plan is going to require a huge increase in both state and federal taxes with no relief in your insurance premiums.

At least we have already demonstrated in this book that by going to a single-payer system, we can improve on the care we currently receive and do it with even fewer dollars than we currently are spending.

The difference between the two plans lies in where the money goes. This country needs affordable health care, not affordable health insurance.

Now, in either system (private or public), in order for it to be successful, participation must be mandatory.

In a single-payer system, that is easy to do. There is only one risk pool. Everyone pays his or her fair share according to ability, and everyone is covered.

Under the AHIP proposal, it's not so easy. There are still gaps. There are still patients who will have poor paying and undesirable coverage plans. Doctors and hospitals will still be forced to play the game of "competitive avoidance" and will still be stuck trying to collect deductibles from patients who can't afford to fund their UHAs. There will still be patients with bare bones coverage plans who can't afford their medications and preventive visits. And, worst of all, there will still be patients "stuck in the middle" who will not be eligible for government programs yet still will be considered uninsurable by private industry.

In a December 31, 2006, *Los Angeles Times* article by Lisa Girion—"Healthy? Insurers don't buy it,"—Ms. Girion tried to address the issue of private insurance "cherry picking" for healthy, low-risk patients (otherwise euphemistically referred to as medical underwriting). She referred to a recent consumer survey that reported 1 in 5 people who applied for health insurance were either denied or charged a higher premium because of pre-existing conditions. (I can tell you from personal experience as a medical director of an HMO that it's a lot higher than that.)

The comments she received from industry spokespersons were revealing, but not surprising. A spokeswoman for PacifiCare Health Systems Inc. said, "Our goal is to extend affordable coverage to as many people as we can, but because of the medical underwriting, we do not accept everybody." Another spokesman for Kaiser Permanente noted that in order for the health maintenance organization to remain solvent, it had to be restrictive—"We have to be very careful to not enroll a bunch of people who are going to spend all the money on their care."

So, in the face of mandatory purchasing, we now face another moral dilemma. If we allow the insurance companies to continue to cherry pick, we will, in essence, give them the green light to dump responsibility for all the high-risk, undesirable patients back on the taxpayers, while they continue to bask in their excessive profits. If we mandate by law that private insurance covers everyone regardless of prior existing conditions (guaranteed issue), this will force the insurance industry to set its premiums based on population risk (community rating). Because each insured pool will have a higher number of high-risk patients, this will, by default, drive up the cost for everyone in the pool, increasing even further the financial burden for the working middle class. In either scenario, the cost of health care will continue its vicious cyclic torrent, while the insurance industry continues to ride the wave of excessive profit taking. Damned if you do and damned if you don't—either way the people lose!

Meanwhile, back to the AHIP plan. Even by its own calculations, the AHIP projects that once this plan is fully implemented, at the end of 10 years we will still have an uninsured rate of 5 percent. That is 15 million Americans who will still have no health insurance! And, worst of all, the administrative costs to doctors and hospitals for trying to keep up with the continued fragmentation of this program will, if anything, go up. (Just before our clinic went under in the fall of 2004, our administrator and I sat down and calculated that 23 percent of our overhead was the amount required to support the administrative staff that was needed to deal with the bureaucracy imposed upon us by the insurance industry. Yes, Medicare and Medicaid had their own issues, but the administrative costs of those programs were nothing compared to the bureaucratic behemoth of the private insurance industry that we had to fight on a daily basis.)

As we pointed out, the poorest and the sickest patients who are the highest risk for consuming the most health care dollars will be funneled over to be covered by the government. Everyone else, one way or the other, will be forced to buy coverage from whom? The insurance industry, of course. And all of those people who sit between Medicaid eligibility and 400 percent of FPL will be forced to buy health insurance, and their premiums will be subsidized with your tax dollars. For most of us in middle class America, not only will we experience a huge tax increase, but we will continue to pay our expensive insurance premiums. And through it all, there is still no mechanism for containing cost.

The insurance industry can avoid the sickest and poorest, shift first dollar costs over to doctors, hospitals, and the lower middle class, and, at the same time, increase its enrollments (and profits) with government money in the form of tax vouchers and subsidies.

What a coup! As we mentioned earlier, one motivation for keeping health care dollars in the private sector is to stimulate innovation. This is one of the most innovative profit-enhancing schemes this country has seen in decades. This is what expanding private enterprise in the financing of health care will get you. Doctors and hospitals have an obligation to provide the best health care they can in the most cost-effective manner possible. They are not always successful, but most are conscientious enough to do their best. On the other hand, for-profit insurance companies have a fiduciary responsibility first and foremost to their shareholders—that is priority one!

Still not convinced? Weiss Ratings Inc., which provides review and investment ratings for stocks and funds as well as financial risk ratings for banks and insurance companies, has shown a most interesting trend since the beginning of the decade. Beginning in 2000, the cumulative earnings of the 500 or so for-profit HMO insurance companies being tracked by Weiss Ratings were nearly $1 billion. Over the next 5 years, this trend would escalate so that by the second quarter of 2005 their earnings exceeded $6.5 billion. The data ends at that point but reflects annualized profits of $13 billion.[6]

Even if you take into account the $1.8 billion the industry lost from 1997-1999, the return on investment is astronomical.

What is even more astonishing is taking into account what happened in that same time frame. Primary care physician real income actually declined by about 5 percent,[7] while the uninsured rate went from 40 to 45 million, and the number of people covered under employer-sponsored insurance fell from 69 to 60 percent.[8]

Yet, from 2000 to the second quarter of 2005 (where the data reporting ends), the cumulative earnings of the for-profit HMO industry increased by 650 percent. If that trend were to continue, on an annualized basis it would be 1,300 percent by year's end![9]

Talk about innovation! Let me introduce you to the fox who wants to guard the henhouse!

Doctors and hospitals need to come together and create more innovative ways to improve the safety and efficiency of health care delivery and do so in a more cost-effective manner. We do not need innovation that creates more efficient ways to improve the profitability of investors whose only interest in health care is making money. And we certainly don't need our tax dollars to light the way into investors' pockets.

The *Los Angeles Times* reported on November 23, 2006,[10] that Cigna Corporation, which has underwritten health insurance for the entertainment industry through its professional associations for 25 years, would be raising its premiums by an average of 82 percent. Premiums on its point-of-service plan will rise to $1,022 per month for single members and $2,485 per month for families. That's $29,820 per year for family coverage! Even with government subsidies, no middle-class American can afford these premiums.

Then one must ask the question, why an 82 percent hike in premiums when health care inflation has "stabilized" at 8 percent?[11] Why? Because they can. Most Americans have no idea what goes on inside this industry.

Dr. William McGuire, former CEO of UnitedHealth Group (one of America's largest and most profitable insurance companies), was featured as one of the highest-paid executives in U.S. history with a salary of $8 million a year with benefits and fully vested stock options exceeding $1.6 billion. Yes, that was billion with a capital "B."

Dr. McGuire resigned from his position as of December 1, 2006, amidst a company scandal and a formal investigation by the Securities and Exchange Commission (SEC) for backdating stock options for executives—an act meant to inflate the portfolios of those at the helm in order "reward" their leadership for excessive company profits. This accounting trick was part of what helped Dr. McGuire to amass his fortune, using your excessive health insurance premiums to get there. UnitedHealth has been working cooperatively with the SEC and promises to rectify any apparent wrongdoing. But even if it must readjust its accounting and is forced to restate its earnings downward covering the period between 1994 and 2005 (with an amount that could be as high as $1.7 billion), the effect on its Wall Street stock prices has been minimal. UnitedHealth still projects an 11 percent increase in revenue with net earnings of $4.7 billion for 2007.[12, 13, 14]

So? Isn't this is just another day at the office for Wall Street and business as usual for corporate America? Yes, it is, and that's the problem! These are the games that are being played every day at the highest echelons of the for-profit insurance industry. While the board of directors for UnitedHealth discusses "certain interpretive issues" on how to restate their earnings for Wall Street, Dr. McGuire is waiting to see if his retirement in stock options is worth a couple of hundred million or one and a half billion dollars. At the same time, thousands of hardworking American families are trying to decide between paying their winter heating bill or dropping their health insurance.

I certainly do not begrudge, nor is it my intent to attack, the hallowed halls of corporate America. But health care is a service industry; we are not manufacturing light poles or trading soybeans with Argentina. These types of corporate games are deadly! While for-profit insurance companies are moving hundreds of billions of dollars from one side of the ledger to other and taking their share of the booty (whether legal or not), in the process millions of Americans are suffering or dying needlessly. All because they can't afford health care.

I will say it again—the for-profit health insurance industry is not in the business of providing quality, affordable, and equitable health care; it is in the business of making money. Its motivation is greed. And as long as greed is allowed to drive health care policy and finance, we will never be able to achieve the common good of a healthy and productive electorate.

Even now, our elected officials are being lobbied by the AMA and AHIP to raise your taxes in order to pump hundreds of billions of additional dollars into a system that promises nothing except to bolster Wall Street and make billionaires of America's health insurance CEOs.

Thankfully, there are some things they can't get away with. But they keep on trying.

An October 31, 2006, *Chicago Tribune* article[15] concerned the story of a recent court case in which Amerigroup Corporation and its subsidiary Amerigroup Illinois was ordered to pay damages of $144 million for discriminating against pregnant women and high-risk patients.

Amerigroup is a private organization that runs managed-care plans and claims it can manage the cost of Medicaid more efficiently than the state through traditional fee-for-service. The organization set corporate policy in place that purposely set up barriers to avoid enrolling pregnant women and potentially high-risk patients. Its policy, according to one executive, was to "go after the healthies."

Of course, not all health insurance executives are crooks, but I could go on for pages with articles about disasters and lawsuits stemming from patients who lost their coverage, had their coverage denied, or ended up losing everything because of technicalities or fine print in an insurance contract.[16] In fact, in one case, a patient was dropped from coverage because the insurance company claimed that the patient failed to report an illness that occurred during childhood.

The insanity has got to stop!

Sadly, it won't stop until we remove greed as the motivation for the financing of health care.

So, what is the alternative? Get rid of insurance companies and move to a national health plan?

We are already two-thirds of the way there. On December 3, 2006, *The New York Times* ran an article by Daniel Gross entitled "National Health Care? We're Halfway There." In it, Gross cited research from some of the most prestigious sources of health care policy, including the Employee Benefits Research Institute; the federal Agency for Healthcare Research and Quality (AHRQ); Uwe Reinhardt, professor of political economics at Princeton; and David Himmelstein, MD, associate professor of medicine at Harvard Medical School.

Sorting through the data of what our government spends on health care, the findings are incredible, and probably most Americans are totally unaware of their significance.

Many politicians claim that if we went to a universal health care system, it would totally drain the economy and bankrupt the country. However, Thomas M. Selden, economist at the AHRQ, points out that the tax subsidy for employment-related coverage was $208 billion in 2006. That amounts to 35.4 percent of the amount spent on private insurance premiums. Also in 2006, federal spending on Medicare was $378 billion, with $180.6 billion on Medicaid. (Remember that the $180.6 billion federal dollars going toward Medicaid is nearly matched with an additional $160 billion in funding from the states.)

Now, when you factor in health spending for the military, the Veterans Administration, Indian Health Services, federal employee benefits, Medicare, Medicaid, and all federal tax subsidies for health care, total federal spending on health care comes to $1.2 trillion for 2006. That equates to over 60 percent of total health care spending as a nation. This does not take into account the tax subsidies and other contributions being offered by the individual states, many of which have their income tax tied to federal returns. Nor does it include the amount of free care being written off by doctors and hospitals that is already being subsidized by the remainder of the system.

Why is this so important?

In December 2006, the Canadian Institute for Health Information released its annual report of health care spending. The report issued the expected increase in spending, health care dollars as a percentage of Gross Domestic Product, etc. But the most striking finding for us to consider is actually the most subtle and overlooked. It is the ratio of public to private shares of total health care spending. The Canadian ratio has been very consistent over the past decade at 70/30.[17]

In other words, the Canadians are able to offer exceptional health care for all of their citizens with the government providing 70 percent of total health care spending.

Right now, the U.S. federal government supplies over 60 percent of total health care spending (not including all the unaccounted dollars on a state-by-state basis). Yet we have one of the worst health care systems in the entire industrialized world with 46 million of our citizens having no coverage.

Our government already has a budget set as if it were providing a national health insurance program. We already have the capacity to offer exceptional health care for everyone in this country without compromising the quality of care that most Americans enjoy, and we can do it without coming up with any more money.

All we have to do is reorganize our current funding mechanisms, unify the administrative process, and remove the profit motive from the financing of health care.

This nation could not function at its current level of production or maintain the level of health it currently enjoys without its doctors and hospitals. But I guarantee that nearly every one of us could wake up some morning in the not-too-distant future and not even notice if the for-profit insurance companies ceased to exist. They are antiquated, unnecessary, and the single biggest stumbling block to the health, welfare, and productivity of our great nation.

So, in closing, how do we make it work?

The three biggest fears of a single-payer system are:

1. Endless waiting lines frequently referred to as the "queue"

2. A faceless, monstrous bureaucracy

3. Rationing

First, we have already shown that we have the money. We have sufficient funds to maintain our infrastructure, for example, CT scans, MRI machines, specialists, etc. Part of the reason why countries like Canada carry the stigma of waiting lines is because they failed to maintain their infrastructure. Most European nations have been very successful in managing the balance between capacity and need. If we fail to maintain our infrastructure, we will have no one to blame but ourselves. Besides, at present the United States has its own perverted form of queue management. It is called: If you can't afford it, you don't get it!

Second, in regard to the faceless, monstrous bureaucracy, let's talk about Medicare for a moment. What is so scary about Medicare? As a physician, I can tell you that it is one of the easiest organizations to deal with, especially on an administrative level. And what about the patients? Have your parents or your grandparents ever said to you, "Gee, I wish I could drop my Medicare and go back on my expensive private insurance." No, never. (Medicare Part D does not count. In fact, the reason why we have had so many problems with Medicare Part D is because we tried to privatize it!) I cannot tell you how many times I have had patients say to me, "Dr. White, I am going to wait until next summer to see the heart specialist, because right now I can't afford my insurance. I go on Medicare next July, and in the meantime I just hope and pray that I don't get any sicker."

To anyone in their late 50s or early 60s, invariably, Medicare is a beacon of hope, not a resignation to socialism. Why can't we offer that beacon of hope to all of our fellow Americans?

Finally, rationing. The dreaded "R" word.

Since the opponents of a single-payer system can no longer wave a communist flag in our faces to convince all good, God-fearing Americans that a national health program is the last step leading to the hammer and sickle flying atop the Capitol, the next scare tactic is the "R" word.

As we alluded to above, this nation already rations care and creates queues. But, unlike the rest of the industrialized nations of the world, we ration not according to the principles of sound science but according to geography, social class, competitive avoidance, and ability to pay.

Don McCanne, a senior health policy fellow and editor of "Quote of the Day," made this comment regarding rationing: "At our level of spending, there would be no need to ration reasonable, beneficial health services, though we should reduce funding for non-beneficial or detrimental services. But that is not rationing; that is called *value purchasing,* a feature of well-functioning health systems."

This nation already spends more health care dollars per capita then any other nation on earth. There is no reason why we cannot establish a not-for-profit national health program without compromising the level of care that those with good insurance now presently enjoy.

Using rationing as an argument against a well-designed single-payer system is a baseless scare tactic and needs to be permanently removed from the rhetoric of debate!

However, I must make one thing perfectly clear. The key to a successful single-payer system lies in its governance. To ensure its success:

1. It must be accountable to the people.

2. Its budget must be insulated from the Legislature.

3. It must be run like a public utility.

What an incredible system it would be if we just gave it a chance!

So how do we create a universally accessible, publicly financed system that is accountable to the people, has the authority to contain excessive health care inflation, uses evidence-based medicine to determine the best value for our health care dollars, and will do it on a democratic platform? Is there such a program?

In fact, there is. In Colorado there is a bill that has not yet been introduced but is gaining momentum and support from many well-respected constituencies that addresses the so-important issue of governance.

This bill calls for the establishment of a state health care funding trust that is separate and insulated from the general funding mechanisms of the Colorado Legislature. It is built on the model of the Federal Reserve and is governed by a Board of Trustees whose time on the board is term-limited and accountable to the people—not appointed by the executive branch.

It basically establishes a single, publicly owned, not-for-profit insurance company governed and administrated as a public utility.

The governing board is given the power to set budgets; standards of care; benefits and limits of coverage; oversight of health-related regulatory agencies and public health; licensure and credentialing; negotiations for the single state formulary; oversight of a malpractice and safety board (which makes the process of malpractice and physician discipline one of education and adjustments within the system, to improve patient safety instead of a purely punitive legal process); and most important, it provides a forum for open debate and public input on thorny issues of ethics, value purchasing, and cost/benefit ratios. This platform can then direct discussion toward ways to improve public health, not the effects they may have on stockholder earnings. And it does so on a democratic platform.

The board is required to hold public meetings and maintain transparency in its governance. In a sense, this is truly consumer-directed health care.

The bill creates five districts within the state so that each district has its own administration and medical director. This allows for the subtle differences that sometimes occur in regions with differing needs and patient populations; for example, asthma-related illness in inner city children is not the same public health concern as machinery-related accidents for farm kids in a rural district.

The financing is provided through a combination of already established state and federal funding by placing Medicare and Medicaid dollars into a single pool. Then, the premiums going into the present multilayered insurance industry are replaced with income tax contributions and mandatory enrollment, thus creating a single risk pool and a single streamlined administrative process. (Centralizing the administrative process alone will shave off between 25 and 30 percent of total health care expenditures simply by eliminating duplicative layers of administration and profit-taking.)

So what about the delivery of and access to health care? As far as consumers are concerned, for most, it will actually improve. The concepts of "preferred providers" and "in- or out-of-network systems" are eliminated. Patients are allowed to see the doctor and hospital of their choice anywhere in the state. If they need to see a doctor in another state, the system pays for that visit up to what is paid within the program and the patient pays the difference, if there is any. Emergency care is covered for out-of-state travel. Medicines and durable medical supplies are part of the coverage.

Regarding doctors and hospitals, nothing changes. Only the financing of health care sits in the public sector. Doctors and hospitals may remain in the private, fee-for-service model. The only difference is that everyone gets paid the same for the same procedure, in effect eliminating "competitive avoidance." An inner city hospital gets the same reimbursement for a Level 1 trauma gunshot wound coming from a homeless shelter as a suburban hospital ER receiving a Level 1 trauma motor vehicle accident involving a corporate executive. And a family doctor in Colorado Springs gets paid the same for a Level 3 office visit as a rural colleague doing checkups out of a mobile clinic in a remote mining town.

The beauty of all this is the doctors and hospitals only have to learn the ropes of one administrative bureaucracy to which they have direct access when problems arise. They only bill one entity, thus eliminating an army of administrators and clerks.

But, best of all, doctors and hospitals can start competing with one another, not on issues of landing the best contracts and avoiding the poorest-paying patients, but where it counts—patient satisfaction, safety, efficacy, and improved clinical outcomes.

That, after all, is why I went to medical school!

And what about the effects on business? I, for the life of me, have the hardest time understanding why so many business owners are so adamantly opposed to the concept of a single-payer system. Although I have come to learn that, for most Americans, it boils down to fear and not fully understanding our current methods of financing. So many business owners tell me that they want to maintain our current system so they can have choice and preserve competition.

We have already presented ample evidence to show that in health care there is no free market, and competition follows the axiom of unintended consequences. And what about having a choice? Do you really have a choice now? Is picking the lesser of two evils considered a realistic choice? Right now, most businesses across this nation are facing only two options—keep health benefits for their employees and struggle or remain competitive and drop health benefits for their employees. What kind of a choice is that?

So let's look at what this Colorado plan could do for business. The program is partially funded through state income and corporate tax deductions, thus removing the sole burden of health benefits from business. However, companies are allowed to make all or part of their employees tax contribution if they so choose.

There are also several hidden benefits that are overlooked:

1. Workers' Compensation: Under the single-payer plan, everyone is already covered. The only workers' compensation that needs to be purchased is disability. Because personal injury and medical bills (which are the lion's share of workers' compensation premiums) are eliminated, business premiums would be dramatically reduced, and the fear of one's premiums going through the roof after an injury are minimized. This also frees up employers to hire individuals who may have had a previous injury without fear of increasing their risk rating.

2. General liability: Again, any business that deals directly with the public, such as a lumberyard, a grocery store, or a municipality with a public park, only needs to cover disability and property damage. General liability premiums would be dramatically reduced.

3. Auto insurance: Again, premiums would be greatly reduced, especially for companies or large farms that have fleets of machinery and operators. This benefit would also extend to individuals, as personal injury medical expenses would be classified as no fault and would not have to be sought after or settled for in the case of litigation.

When business begins to add up the insurance savings, along with the added benefit of a simplified and more efficient personnel benefits department (not to mention a healthier, more productive work force), U.S. companies can finally start concentrating on what they do best: marketing American-made products with a competitive edge, in both domestic and international markets.

But Dr. White, won't we lose the advantage of innovative competition by removing the insurance companies and establishing a public monopoly on the financing of health care?

That's what this book is all about. We have established the fact that there is no effective way to deliver quality, affordable, and equally accessible care with private sector financing. It can't be done. We are attempting to promote the health and productivity of our nation. We are not making widgets.

Finally, I will leave you with one last thought. Health care is a service industry meant for the greater good. Tonight after you have retired this book to the shelf, I want you to go to a quiet place and think about what would happen to your community if your local fire and police departments were converted to for-profit, fee-for-service industries. Imagine them being financed with a combination of poorly funded public support, depending heavily on fee-for-service reimbursement (or bribery) from people who may or may not have the funds to afford their service. Think of the chaos, the inequality, the unnecessary loss of life, the injustice, and the potential for abuse. Think about entire neighborhoods of lower income individuals or remote rural areas with no fire or police protection at all, because they are deemed "unprofitable."

Privatization of these services is unconscionable!

Now think about our health care system. Why should medicine be any different?

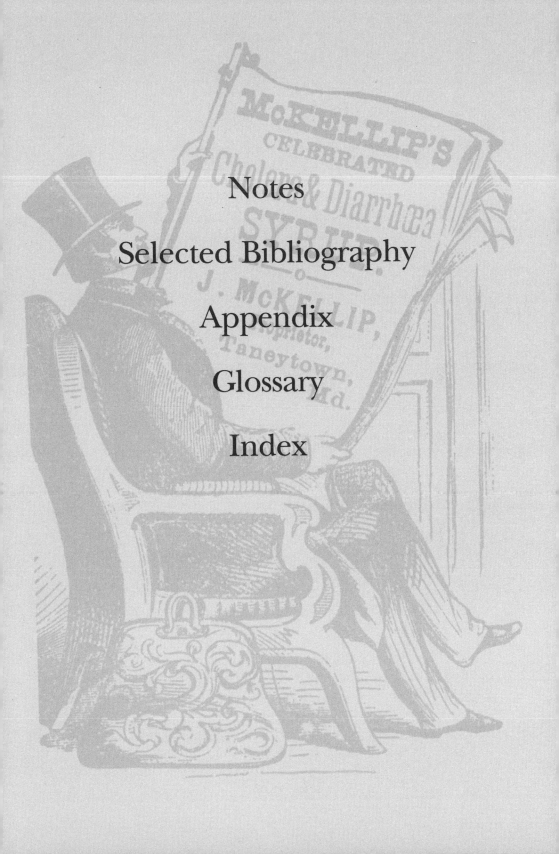

Notes

Selected Bibliography

Appendix

Glossary

Index

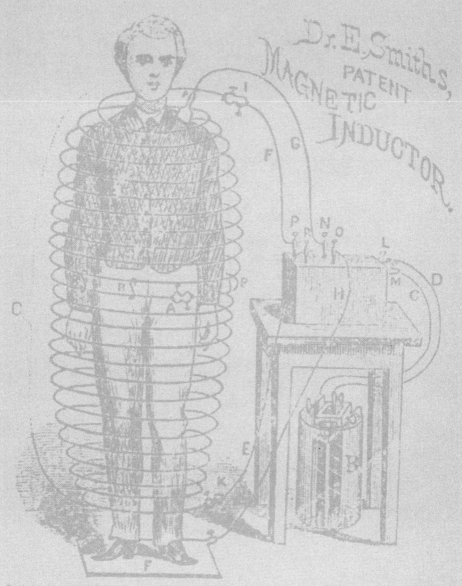

Dr. E. Smith's,
PATENT
MAGNETIC
INDUCTOR.

Notes

INTRODUCTION

1. See: <www.coveringtheuninsured.org>

2. Health economist Uwe Reinhardt used this term when he described what some parents were forced to become in order to get care for their children in: Uwe E. Reinhardt, PhD, "Wanted: A Clearly Articulated Social Ethic for American Health Care," *JAMA* 278 (17) November 5, 1997:1446-1447.

3. Former Senator Bob Kerrey's testimony before the Senate Finance Committee on "The Administration's FY 2003 Budget Proposals for Prescription Drugs," March 7, 2002.

CHAPTER 1

1. Stephen Bezruchka, MD, "Is Our Society Making You Sick?" *Newsweek,* February 26, 2001, p. 14.

2. Barbara Starfield, MD, MPH, "Is U.S. Health Care Really the Best in the World?" *JAMA* 284 (4) October 25, 2000: 483-485.

3. World Health Organization, *The World Health Report 2000. Health Systems: Improving Performance,* Geneva, 2000.

4. "Emergency Care 'Safety Net' Unraveling," *USA Today*, February 4-6, 2000.

5. Available at <www.acponline.org/uninsured/>

6. Kaiser Family Foundation, "Sicker and Poorer: The Consequences of Being Uninsured," May 2002 <www.kff.org>

7. Institute of Medicine, *Care Without Coverage: Too Little, Too Late*, National Academy Press, 2002.

8. Richard F. Corlin, MD, "The Time Is Right to Fix the Problem of the Uninsured," *American Medical News,* January 21, 2002.

9. See: Kevin Grumbach, MD, "Insuring the Uninsured. Time to End the Aura of Invisibility," *JAMA* 284 (16) October 25, 2000: 2114-2116.

10. Jane Bryant Quinn, "The Invisible Uninsured," *Newsweek,* March 1, 1999.

11. Laurie Garrett, *Betrayal of Trust: The Collapse of Global Public Health,* Hyperion, New York, 2000.

12. J. D. Kleinke, *Oxymorons: The Myth of the U.S. Health Care System,* Jossey-Bass, 2001.

13. Personal communication, December 13, 2001.

14. Our Community Health Center serves a total of about 18,000 patients in southwest Idaho. Our staff includes eight physicians and eight mid-levels (nurse practitioners and physician assistants). We have a large number of patients with diabetes because our population is about half Hispanic.

15. World Health Organization, *"The World Health Report, 2006."*

16. Office of the Actuary, Centers for Medicare & Medicaid Services, 2006.

17. Donald W. Light, "Health Care for All: A Conservative Case," *Commonweal*, February 22, 2002.

18. Pat Armstrong and Hugh Armstrong, with Claudia Fegan, MD, *Universal Health Care. What the United States Can Learn from the Canadian Experience*, The New Press, New York, 1998.

19. Personal communication from health economist Donald W. Light through "Quote of the Day," March 2002. Available through <www.pnhp.org>

20. Ibid., May 5, 2002.

21. Irene Wielawski, "Gouging the Medically Uninsured: A Tale of Two Bills," *Health Affairs* 19 (5) September/October 2000: 180-185.

22. See: <www.kff.org>

23. Henry J. Kaiser Family Foundation, "Prescription Drug Trends," Washington, D.C., July 2000.

24. Center for Policy Alternatives, "Prescription Drugs Policy Toolkit."

25. U.S. Department of Health and Human Services, "Securing the Benefits of Medical Innovation for Seniors: The Role of Prescription Drugs and Drug Coverage," July 2002. <aspe.hhs.gov/health/reports/medicalinnovation/> The report defends the pricing and profits of U.S. drug manufacturers.

26. Shannon Little, "Public Citizen Report Debunks R&D Myths," *Public Citizen News*, September/October 2001.

27. This phenomenon is described in an article by Jeff Gerth and Sheryl Gay Stolberg, "Drug Companies Profit From Research Supported by Taxpayers," *The New York Times*, April 23, 2000.

28. The Associated Press, "States: Drug Maker Delayed Generics," *The Idaho Statesman*, June 5, 2002. Taxol was discovered by the National Cancer Institute, which licensed the drug to Bristol-Myers.

29. Sheryl Gay Stolberg and Jeff Gerth, "How Companies Stall Generics and Keep Themselves Healthy," *The New York Times*, July 23, 2000.

30. A similar situation exists for the middlemen who do group purchasing of medical supplies for hospitals. See Chapter 2, "Ignorance of the Costs."

31. For accounts of these practices, see: <www.nofreelunch.org> and Rudolph J. Mueller, MD, *As Sick As It Gets*, Olin Frederick, Inc., Dunkirk, NY, 2001, Chapter 4, "The Pharmaceutical Companies."

32. Marcia Angell, MD, "The Pharmaceutical Industry—To Whom Is It Accountable?" *New England Journal of Medicine* 342 (25) June 22, 2000: 1902-1904.

33. Karen Davis, "Universal Coverage in the United States: Lessons from Experience of the 20th Century," *Journal of Urban Health: Bulletin of the New York Academy of Medicine* 78 March 2001: 46-58.

34. Mahyar Mofidi, DMD, MPH; R. Gary Rozier, DDS, MPH; and Rebecca S. King, DDS, MPH, "Problems With Access to Care for Medicaid-Insured Children: What Caregivers Think," *American Journal of Public Health* 92 (1) January 2002: 53.

35. Sara Rosenbaum, JD, "Medicaid," *New England Journal of Medicine* 346 February 21, 2002: 635-640.

36. Robert Pear, "9 of 10 Nursing Homes in U.S. Lack Adequate Staff, a Government Study Finds," *The New York Times*, February 18, 2002.

37. Uwe E. Reinhardt, PhD, in a speech before the National Chamber of Commerce, October 1999.

38. David Broder, "Fix Health Care Now," *The Washington Post*, January 6, 2002, Op-ed.

39. Molly Ivins, Creators Syndicate, Inc. column, March 26, 2002. Ivins adds, "But if you want to see horror in action, try the emergency room of any large public hospital in this country."

CHAPTER 2

1. Elaborating on her "passion" for solving the problem of the uninsured, Ms. Cohen was speaking on a panel that took place on April 30, 2002, to discuss House Concurrent Resolution 99, the "Health Care Access Resolution." Ms. Cohen was one of the chief architects of New York's Family Health Plus Program.

2. *Des Moines Register* Editorial Board, "The Health-Care Hodgepodge. A Single-Payer National Plan Makes More and More Sense," *The Des Moines Register*, January 4, 2002, Editorial section.

3. Rudolph J. Mueller, MD, *As Sick As It Gets*, Olin Frederick, Inc., Dunkirk, NY, 2001.

4. Kathleen O'Connor, MA, *The Buck Stops Nowhere: Why America's Healthcare Is All Dollars and No Sense*, Hara Publishing Company, Seattle, 2001.

5. Richard G. A. Feachem et al., "Getting More for Their Dollar: A Comparison of the NHS With California's Kaiser Permanente," *British Medical Journal* 324 January 25, 2002: 135-143.

6. However, as Grumbach points out, the British health care system spends less than one-third per capita than the U.S. system, and ". . . for macrolevel economic efficiency, the NHS remains the standard bearer."

7. Uwe E. Reinhardt, PhD, "Harness Information to Make Health Care Work," *Managed Care*, January 2002. He says, "From the perspective of those who pay for health care and of those who use it, our system remains one of the most opaque sectors in the economy."

8. Vicki Lankarge, for insure.com. Posted on *MSN Money*, February 6, 2002.

9. Walt Bogdanich, "2 Powerful Groups Hold Sway Over Buying at Many Hospitals," *The New York Times*, March 4, 2002.

10. Sherry A. Glied, "Challenges and Options for Increasing the Number of Americans With Health Insurance," The Commonwealth Fund, January 2001, p. 13.

11. Donald W. Light, "Health Care for All: A Conservative Case," *Commonweal*, February 22, 2002.

12. Malcolm K. Sparrow, *License to Steal: How Fraud Bleeds America's Health Care System*, Westview Press, 2000.

13. S. M. Asch, E. M. Sloss, G. Hogan, R. H. Brook, and R. L. Kravitz, "Measuring Underuse of Necessary Care Among Elderly Medicare Beneficiaries Using Inpatient and Outpatient Claims," *JAMA* 284 (2000): 2325-33.

14. Figures from OECD data from 1996. Gerard Anderson and Peter Sotir Hussey, "Comparing Health System Performance in OECD Countries," *Health Affairs*, May/June 2001.

CHAPTER 3

1. Ironically, another new expensive rheumatoid arthritis drug, which was pulled from the market because of its harmful side effects, has caused one pharmaceutical manufacturer to be taken to court, costing it millions of dollars and severe damage to its reputation.

2. See: Steven J. Katz et al., "Phantoms in the Snow: Canadians' Use of Health Care Services in the United States," *Health Affairs* 21 (3) May/ June 2002: 19-31. In this 1996 study, only 20 of 18,000 respondents said they had purposefully gone to the United States to obtain any kind of health care.

3. Gordon Brown, Chancellor of the Exchequer, *The Economist*, April 13-18, 2002, p. 18.

4. Rema Cohen, speaking as a panelist on a discussion of House Concurrent Resolution 99, the "Health Care Access Resolution," April 30, 2002.

5. Julie Appleby, "Hospitals Fight for Turf in Medical Arms Race," *USA Today*, February 20, 2002.

6. Michael J. Mandel, "Economic Trends: Health Care's Economic Payoff," *Business Week*, April 29, 2002.

7. Michael Freedman, "The Tort Mess," *Forbes*, May 13, 2002, pp. 91-98.

8. Joseph Anthony, "The Answer for Small Business: Guaranteed Health Care," December 2001, <www.bcentral.com/articles/anthony/166.asp>

9. Robert Kuttner, "A Dirty Little Secret: Managed Care Is Bad for Business," *Business Week*, December 21, 1998, p. 18.

10. Mike Wallace, "Mind and Body," *The New York Times*, December 11, 2001, Op-ed.

11. Paul M. Ellwood, Jr., MD, "Does Managed Care Need to Be Replaced?" *Medscape General Medicine*, October 22, 2001.

12. Ibid.

13. Office of the Actuary, Centers for Medicare & Medicaid Services, 2006.

14. COBRA guarantees some employees continuation of their insurance coverage for 18 months after leaving their jobs, but the employee must pay for the coverage.

CHAPTER 4

1. Drew Altman, "The Uninsured Find Fewer Doctors in the House," *The New York Times*, August 30, 1998.

2. See: American College of Physicians-American Society of Internal Medicine, "No Health Insurance? It's Enough to Make You Sick— Scientific Research Linking the Lack of Health Coverage to Poor Health," 2000, <www.acponline.org/uninsured/lack-contents.htm> and Kaiser Family Foundation, "Sicker and Poorer: The Consequences of Being Uninsured," May 2002, <www.kff.org>

3. Edward W. Gregg et al., "Use of Diabetes Preventive Care and Complications Risk in Two African-American Communities," *American Journal of Preventive Medicine* 21 (3) October 2001: 197-202.

4. Bob Herbert, "Hunger in the City," *The New York Times*, November 22, 2001, Op-ed.

CHAPTER 5

1. "Second Class Medicine," *Consumer Reports*, September 2000, pp. 42-50.

2. Robert L. Ferrer, MD, MPH, "A Piece of My Mind. Within the System of No-System," *JAMA* 286 (20) November 28, 2001: 2513-2514.

3. In 2002, 200 percent of poverty was $36,200 for a family of four.

4. John Holahan and Brenda Spillman, "Health Care Access for Uninsured Adults: A Strong Safety Net Is Not the Same as Insurance," The Urban Institute, Series B, No. B-42, January 2002.

CHAPTER 6

1. M. Edith Rasell, MD, "Cost Sharing in Health Insurance—a Reexamination," *New England Journal of Medicine* 332 (17) April 27, 1995.

2. R. G. Evans, M. L. Barer, and C. Hertzman, "The 20-year Experiment: Accounting for, Explaining, and Evaluating Health Care Cost Containment in Canada and the United States," *Annual Review of Public Health* 12 (1991): 481-518.

3. R. Tamblyn, R. Laprise, J. A. Hanley et al., "Adverse Events Associated With Prescription Drug-Cost Sharing Among Poor and Elderly Persons," *JAMA* 285 (2001): 421-429.

4. That is, insurance that paid everything with zero co-pays and deductibles.

CHAPTER 7

No notes.

CHAPTER 8

1. For a complete discussion of the issue, see: Laurie Garrett, *Betrayal of Trust: The Collapse of Global Public Health*, Hyperion, New York, 2000.

2. Gerald P. Balcar and Rudolph J. Mueller, MD, *Inside the American Healthcare Crisis: The Causes, the Economics, the Treatment*, Olin Frederick, Inc., Dunkirk, NY, 2004.

3. Campaign for Children's Health Care, *"No Shelter from the Storm: America's Uninsured Children,"* Publication CCHC-0601, September 2006.

CHAPTER 9

1. James Dao, "On the Streets of Baltimore, the Word on Medicare Is 'Expand,' Not 'Reform,' " *The New York Times*, September 8, 2000.

2. Economic Policy Institute, *Paycheck Economics*, "Medicare at the Crossroads: Vouchers Take Us in the Wrong Direction," March 2001.

3. Paul Krugman, "Bad Medicine," *The New York Times*, March 19, 2002, Op-ed.

CHAPTER 10

1. David B. Williams, professor of sociology at the University of Michigan, as quoted in *The New York Times*, March 21, 2002. He was reporting on an Institute of Medicine study showing that minorities, even if they're insured, get inferior care in America. He added, ". . . This report demonstrates that the playing field [in American health care] clearly is not level."

2. Julie A. Jacob, "Managed Care Looks Abroad," *American Medical News*, September 6, 1999.

3. World Health Organization, *"The World Health Report, 2006."*

4. Donald W. Light, "Health Care for All: A Conservative Case," *Commonweal*, February 22, 2002.

5. William H. Barker, *Adding Life to Years: Organized Geriatrics Services in Great Britain and Implications for the United States*, The Johns Hopkins University Press, Baltimore and London, 1987.

6. Randi Hutter Epstein, "So Lucky to Give Birth in England," *The New York Times*, December 4, 2001, Health & Fitness section.

7. See: Steven J. Katz et al., "Phantoms in the Snow: Canadians' Use of Health Care Services in the United States," *Health Affairs* 21 (3) May/ June 2002: 19-31. In this study, the myth of the "droves" of Canadians coming south for health care is soundly debunked. Only 20 of 18,000 respondents said they had gone to the United States for the purpose of obtaining any type of health care.

8. Pat Armstrong and Hugh Armstrong, with Claudia Fegan, MD, *Universal Health Care. What the United States Can Learn from the Canadian Experience*, The New Press, New York, 1998.

CHAPTER 11

1. "The Unraveling of Health Insurance," *Consumer Reports*, July 2002, pp. 48-53.

2. In the past, as in the '90s, estimates of future health care costs have been fraught with error.

3. See: Michael J. Mandel, "Economic Trends: Health Care's Economic Payoff," *Business Week*, April 29, 2002.

4. See: <www.ahrq.gov>

5. Jonathan P. Weiner, DrPH, "Something 'Nice' Can Come Out of This," *Managed Care*, January 2002.

6. Personal communication. E-mail exchange on PNHP's "Quote of the Day" (August 9, 2001). In Dr. Reinhardt's words: "The real explanation is that the American people prefer a health system whose costs rise in the high double digits. They fought for it at the job and in the political forum. Now they have it. Mazel tov!"

7. David Callahan, *False Hopes: Why America's Quest for Perfect Health Is a Recipe for Failure*, Simon & Schuster, New York, 1998.

8. *The Oregonian*, December 20, 2001. Brandy's surgery, however, was to be covered by private funds raised with the help of a rich benefactor.

9. David Leonhardt, "Health Care As Main Engine: Is That So Bad?" *The New York Times*, November 11, 2001, Money & Business section.

CHAPTER 12

1. Rep. John Conyers, speaking before a panel discussing House Concurrent Resolution 99, the "Health Care Access Resolution," April 30, 2002.

2. Rep. Donna Christian-Christensen, speaking before a panel discussing House Concurrent Resolution 99, the "Health Care Access Resolution," April 30, 2002.

3. R. Michels et al., "Views of Managed Care," *New England Journal of Medicine* 340 (12) March 25,1999: 928.

4. Robert Putnam, "A Better Society in a Time of War," *The New York Times*, October 19, 2001, Op-ed.

CHAPTER 13

1. Richard F. Corlin, MD, as quoted in the *Cedar Rapids Gazette*, April 19, 2002.

2. See: Norbert Goldfield, MD, *National Health Care Reform American Style: Lessons from the Past; A Twentieth Century Journey*, American College of Physician Executives, 2000.

3. Molly Ivins, "Health Care Rx: Phase Out the Failing For-Profit System," *Boulder Daily Camera*, March 28, 2002.

CHAPTER 14

1. Joel E. Miller, "A Perfect Storm: The Confluence of Forces Affecting Health Care Coverage," National Coalition on Health Care, November 2001.

2. Marsha Shuler, "Breaux Favors Health Aid. Senator Backs Universal Coverage for All U.S. Citizens," *The Advocate Online*, January 3, 2002.

3. See: <www.coveringtheuninsured.org>. The organizations include the U.S. Chamber of Commerce, the AFL-CIO, the Business Roundtable, the SEIU (Service Employees International Union), the American Medical Association, the American Nurses Association, the HIAA, Families USA, the American Hospital Association, the Federation of American Hospitals, the Catholic Health Association of the U.S., AARP, and the Robert Wood Johnson Foundation.

4. Pam Belluck, "Small Vote for Universal Care Is Seen as Carrying a Lot of Weight," *The New York Times*, November 16, 2001.

5. As an example, the coveringtheuninsured.org campaign is trying to educate the public about how the uninsured do poorly, die more frequently, and go bankrupt from medical bills. They also have publicized how 80 percent of the uninsured are in working families.

6. For a discussion of the possible role of civil disobedience in health care reform, see: Norbert Goldfield, MD, *National Health Care Reform American Style: Lessons from the Past; A Twentieth Century Journey*, American College of Physician Executives, 2000.

CHAPTER 15

1. Jack A. Meyer and Elliott K. Wicks, "Covering America: Real Remedies for the Uninsured," Economic and Social Research Institute, June 2001.

2. Economic Policy Institute, *Paycheck Economics*, "Medicare at the Crossroads: Vouchers Take Us in the Wrong Direction," March 2001.

3. See: <www.coveringtheuninsured.org>

4. Karen Scott Collins et al., "Diverse Communities, Common Concerns: Assessing Health Care Quality for Minority Americans." See: <www.cmwf.org>

5. R. Michels et al., "Views of Managed Care," *New England Journal of Medicine* 340 (12) March 25, 1999: 928.

6. David Himmelstein and Steffie Woolhandler, *Bleeding the Patient*, Common Courage Press, Monroe, ME, 2001, p. 159.

7. Joel E. Miller, "A Perfect Storm: The Confluence of Forces Affecting Health Care Coverage," National Coalition on Health Care, November 2001.

CHAPTER 16

1. MSNBC's Web site carried an opinion piece from Art Caplan in September 2001 in which Art drew attention to the plight of the uninsured. He advocated for universal coverage, and doing it soon, through the use of government vouchers. This chapter responds to Art's assertion that "Single payer will not fly." My purpose is not so much to disagree with Art as to discuss the political, economic, and ethical relevance of universal coverage with a single-payer-type approach. As explained in this chapter, approaches such as government vouchers are quick fixes, which would only make our already chaotic system more chaotic.

CHAPTER 17

1. "Study Finds Each Pack of Smokes Costs Nation $7 in Care," *The Oregonian*, April 12, 2002.

2. Marie C. Reed and Ha T. Tu, "Triple Jeopardy: Low Income, Chronically Ill, and Uninsured," Issue Brief No. 49, Center for Studying Health Care System Change, February 2002.

3. William C. Knowler et al., "Reduction in the Incidence of Type 2 Diabetes With Lifestyle Intervention or Metformin," *New England Journal of Medicine* 346 (6) February 7, 2002: 393-403.

4. Ali H. Mokdad, PhD, et al., "The Continuing Epidemics of Obesity and Diabetes in the United States," *JAMA* 286 (10) September 10, 2001: 1195-1200.

5. Organisation for Economic Co-operation and Development (OECD), "Health at a Glance," Paris, 2001. For people over 15 years old, the figures show that 25.1 percent of American females (and 19.9 percent of American males) have a BMI over 30. Both are much higher than the numbers for the other 23 countries.

6. Efforts to expel fast food from schools are happening around the country. Texas and California (among other places) are moving to ban junk foods from schools. On the national front, there is Congressional action with the Obesity Prevention and Treatment Act, introduced in May 2002. See: Timothy Egan, "In a Bid to Improve Nutrition, Schools Expel Soda and Chips," *The New York Times*, May 20, 2002.

7. For a more complete discussion of what has happened to food in America, see: (1) Marion Nestle, PhD, MPH, *Food Politics: How the Food Industry Influences Nutrition and Health*, University of California Press, 2002; and (2) Eric Schlosser, *Fast Food Nation: The Dark Side of the All-American Meal*, Houghton Mifflin, 2001.

8. A comprehensive list of policy recommendations to reduce the prevalence of obesity (as well as ideas to promote physical activity) appears in: Marion Nestle, PhD, MPH, and Michael F. Jacobson, PhD, "Halting the Obesity Epidemic: A Public Health Approach," *Public Health Reports* 115 (January/February 2000). Also, the CDC's October 26, 2001, issue of *MMWR (Morbidity and Mortality Weekly Report)*, entitled "Increasing Physical Activity: A Report on Recommendations of the Task Force on Community Preventive Services," is devoted to an analysis of the options for promoting physical activity.

CHAPTER 18

1. An Institute of Medicine study released in March 2002 documented that minorities in America "receive lower quality health care than whites, even when their insurance and income are the same." From *The New York Times*, March 21, 2002.

2. Barbara Ehrenreich, *Nickel and Dimed: On (Not) Getting By in America*, Metropolitan Books, Henry Holt and Company, New York, 2001.

3. Ibid.

CONCLUSION

1. Albert S. Lyons, MD, and R. Joseph Petrucelli II, MD, *Medicine: An Illustrated History*, Abradale Press, Harry N. Abrams, Inc., Publishers, New York, 1987.

2. America's Health Insurance Plans, "We Believe: A Vision for Reform," <www.ahipbelieves.com>

3. Daniel Gross, "National Health Care? We're Halfway There," *The New York Times*, December 3, 2006.

4. Jessica S. Banthin, PhD, and Didem M. Bernard, PhD, "Changes in Financial Burdens for Health Care: National Estimates for the Population Younger Than 65 Years, 1996 to 2003," *JAMA* 296 December 13, 2006: 2712-2719.

5. Sara R. Collins and Jennifer L. Kriss et al., "Squeezed: Why Rising Exposure to Health Care Costs Threatens the Health and Financial Well-Being of American Families," *The Commonwealth Fund*, September 2006.

6. Weiss Ratings Inc. See: <www.weissratings.com>

7. Ha T. Tu and Paul B. Ginsburg, "Losing Ground: Physician Income, 1995-2003," Tracking Report No. 15, Center for Studying Health System Change, June 2006.

8. Kaiser Family Foundation and Health Research and Educational Trust, "Employer Health Benefits—2006 Summary of Findings," 2006.

9. Weiss Ratings Inc. See: <www.weissratings.com>

10. Lisa Girion, "Health premiums to soar for entertainers," *Los Angeles Times*, November 23, 2006.

11. Paul B. Ginsburg, Bradley C. Strunk, Michelle I. Banker, and John P. Cookson, "Tracking Health Care Costs: Spending Growth Remains Stable at High Rate in 2005," Center for Studying Health System Change, Data Bulletin No. 33, October 2006.

12. George Anders, "As Patients, Doctors Feel Pinch, Insurer's CEO Makes a Billion," *Wall Street Journal*, April 18, 2006.

13. Associated Press, "New CEO Takes the Helm at UnitedHealth," December 1, 2006.

14. David Phelps, "UnitedHealth Shares Rise on 2007 Outlook," *Minneapolis-St. Paul Star Tribune*, December 19, 2006.

15. Rudolph Bush, "Jury Finds HMO Bias in Signing Patients," *Chicago Tribune*, October 31, 2006.

16. Lisa Girion, "Kaiser Told to Reinstate Coverage," *Los Angeles Times*, October 19, 2006.

17. Canadian Institute for Health, "Annual Report on Health Care Spending," December 5, 2006.

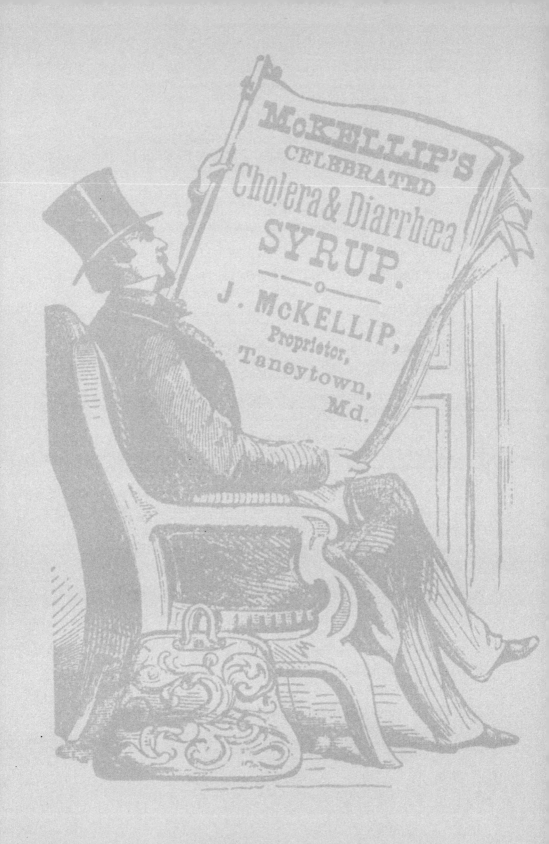

Selected Bibliography

Keeping Up to Date on Health Care Reform

The Kaiser Daily Health Policy Report
    <www.kaisernetwork.org/daily_reports/rep_hpolicy.cfm>

Kaiser Family Foundation Web site: <www.kff.org>

The Commonwealth Fund Web site: <www.cmwf.org>

Physicians for a National Health Program Web site: <www.pnhp.org>

Breaking news Web site: <www.everybodyinnobodyout.org>

American Medical News: <www.amednews.com>

Comprehensive Analysis and Data on the U.S. Health Care System

(These sources include a comprehensive overview of health care policy and cover the full range of topics that are listed separately below.)

Bodenheimer, Thomas S., MD, and Kevin Grumbach, MD.
    Understanding Health Policy. A Clinical Approach. 3rd ed. Lange
    Medical Books. McGraw-Hill, 2002.

Geyman, John P., MD. *Health Care in America: Can Our Ailing
    System Be Healed?* Butterworth/Heinemann, 2002.

Himmelstein, David, MD; Steffie Woolhandler, MD, MPH; and Ida
    Hellander, MD. *Bleeding the Patient.* Monroe, ME: Common
    Courage Press, 2001.

Institute of Medicine Web site: <www.iom.edu/>

Kaiser Family Foundation. "Trends and Indicators in the Changing
    Health Care Marketplace 2002. Chartbook. May 2002. See:
    <www.kff.org>

Kaiser Family Foundation Web site: <www.kff.org>

Mueller, Rudolph J., MD. *As Sick as It Gets.* Dunkirk, NY: Olin
    Frederick, Inc., 2001.

293

Health Care Policy

Angell, Marcia, MD. "Patients' Rights Bills and Other Futile
    Gestures." *New England Journal of Medicine* 342 (22) (June 1,
    2000): 1663-64.

Garrett, Laurie. *Betrayal of Trust: The Collapse of Global Public
    Health.* New York: Hyperion, 2000.

Kleinke, J. D. *Oxymorons: The Myth of the U.S. Health Care System.*
    Jossey-Bass, 2001.

McCanne, Don, MD. "Why Incremental Reforms Will Not Solve the
    Health Care Crisis." *The Journal of the American Board of Family
    Practice* 16 (2003): 257-61.
    <www.jabfp.org/cgi/content/full/16/3/257>

McDonough, John E., DrPH. *Healthcare Policy. The Basics.* The
    Access Project. 1999.

Miller, Joel E. "A Perfect Storm: The Confluence of Forces Affecting
    Health Care Coverage." National Coalition on Health Care.
    November 2001.

Oberlander, Jonathan B., and Theodore R. Marmor. "The Path to
    Universal Health Care." Washington, D. C.: Campaign for
    America's Future, 2000.

O'Connor, Kathleen, MA. *The Buck Stops Nowhere. Why America's
    Healthcare Is All Dollars and No Sense.* Seattle: Hara Publishing
    Group, April 2001.

The Uninsured

American College of Physicians-American Society of Internal
    Medicine. "No Health Insurance? It's Enough to Make You
    Sick—Scientific Research Linking the Lack of Health Coverage
    to Poor Health." 2000. Available at: <www.acponline.org/unin-
    sured/>

Ayanian, John Z., MD, MPP, et al. "Unmet Health Needs of Uninsured
    Adults in the United States." *JAMA* 284 (16) (October 25, 2000):
    2061-69.

Bell, Howard. "Life Without Insurance: True Stories of Unnecessary
    Sickness, Death and Humiliation." *The New Physician* (AMSA).
    September 2000.

Bodenheimer, Thomas, MD, MPH. "Underinsurance in America." *New England Journal of Medicine* 327 (4) (July 23, 1992): 274-78.

Commonwealth Fund Web site: <www.cmwf.org>

Ferrer, Robert L., MD, MPH. "A Piece of My Mind. Within the System of No-System." *JAMA* 286 (20) (November 28, 2001): 2513-14.

Franks, Peter, MD; Carolyn M. Clancy, MD; and Marthe R. Gold, MPH. "Health Insurance and Mortality." *JAMA* 270 (6) (August 11, 1993): 737-41.

Geyman, John P., MD. *Falling Through the Safety Net: Americans Without Health Insurance.* Monroe, ME: Common Courage Press, 2005.

Grumbach, Kevin, MD. "Insuring the Uninsured. Time to End the Aura of Invisibility." *JAMA* 284 (16) (October 25, 2000): 2114-16.

Institute of Medicine. *Care Without Coverage: Too Little, Too Late.* Washington, D. C.: National Academy Press, May 2002.

Kaiser Family Foundation. Commission on Medicaid and the Uninsured. "Covering the Uninsured—Growing Need, Strained Resources." November 2005.

Kaiser Family Foundation. Commission on Medicaid and the Uninsured. "Sicker and Poorer: The Consequences of Being Uninsured." May 2002. <www.kff.org>

Reed, Marie C., and Ha T. Tu. "Triple Jeopardy: Low Income, Chronically Ill, and Uninsured in America." Issue Brief No. 49. Center for Studying Health System Change. February 2002. <www.hschange.org>

Rowland, Diane, ScD. The Kaiser Commission on Medicaid and the Uninsured. "The New Challenge of the Uninsured: Coverage in the Current Economy." Testimony for the Uninsured and Affordable Health Care Coverage Subcommittee on Health. Committee on Energy and Commerce. U.S. House of Representatives. February 28, 2002. <www.kff.org>

"Second-Class Medicine." *Consumer Reports*, September 2000, pp. 42-50.

U. S. Census Bureau, August 2006. "Current Population Reports: Income, Poverty, and Health Insurance Coverage in the United States, 2005."

Safety Net

Caplan, Art, PhD. "New World Calls for New Health Care. Government Should Provide Safety Net for All Americans." September 28, 2001. <www.msnbc.com/news/635352>

Cunningham, P. J., and J. H. May. "A Growing Hole in the Safety Net: Physician Charity Care Drops Again." Tracking Report No. 13. Washington, D.C.: Center for Studying Health System Change, March 2006.

Geyman, John P., MD. *Falling Through the Safety Net: Americans Without Health Insurance*. Monroe, ME: Common Courage Press, 2005.

Kaiser Family Foundation. Commission on Medicaid and the Uninsured Web site. "Addressing the Health Care Impact of Hurricane Katrina, September 15, 2005." Available at <http://www.kff.org/katrina/index.cfm> (accessed September 17, 2005).

Rosenblatt R. A., C. H. Andrilla, T. Curtin, and L. G. Hart. "Shortages of Medical Personnel at Community Health Centers: Implications for Planned Expansion." *JAMA* 295 (2006): 1042-49.

Schiff, G., MD, and C. Fegan, MD. "Community Health Centers and the Underserved: Eliminating Disparities or Increasing Despair?" *Journal of Health Policy* 24 (3/4) (2004): 45-7.

History of Health Care Reform in America

Davis, Karen. "Universal Coverage in the United States: Lessons From Experience of the 20th Century." *Journal of Urban Health: Bulletin of the New York Academy of Medicine* 78 (March 2001): 46-58.

Goldfield, Norbert, MD. *National Health Care Reform American Style: Lessons from the Past; A Twentieth Century Journey*. American College of Physician Executives, 2000.

Oberlander, J. *The Political Life of Medicare*. Chicago: University of Chicago Press, 2003.

Sigerist, H. E. "Medical Care for All the People." *Canadian Journal of Public Health* 35 (7) (1944): 258.

Starr, P. *The Social Transformation of American Medicine*. New York: Basic Books, 1982, pp. 252-53.

Proposals for Health Care Reform

American Academy of Family Physicians. "Assuring Health Care Coverage for All." October 2001. See: <www.aafp.org/unicov/hccfa.pdf>

American College of Physicians-American Society of Internal Medicine. "Achieving Affordable Health Insurance for All Within Seven Years." April 9, 2002. See: <www.acponline.org/hpp/afford—7years.pdf>

Angell, Marcia, MD. "Dispelling the Myths About Single-Payer Health Care." Newsletter of the Universal Health Care Education Fund. November 2001.

Bodenheimer, T. S., MD. The Movement for Universal Health Insurance: Finding Common Ground. *American Journal of Public Health* 93 (2003): 112.

California Health Care Options Project. 2002. Preliminary full drafts of each proposal are available at <http://www.healthcareoptions.ca.gov/doclib.asp>

Caplan, Art, PhD. "New World Calls for New Health Care. Government Should Provide Safety Net for All Americans." September 28, 2001. <www.msnbc.com/news/635352>

Commonwealth Fund Web site: <www.cmwf.org>

Davis, Karen, PhD; Cathy Schoen, MS; and Stephen C. Schoenbaum, MD, MPH. "A 2020 Vision for American Health Care." *Archives of Internal Medicine* 160 (22) (December 11/25, 2000).

Economic Policy Institute. *Paycheck Economics.* "Medicare at the Crossroads: Vouchers Take Us in the Wrong Direction." March 2001.

Evans, R. G. "Going for the Gold: The Redistributive Agenda Behind Market-Based Health Care Reform." *Journal of Health Politics, Policy and Law* 22 (2) (1997): 427.

General Accountability Office (GAO). Federal Employees Benefit Program. "First-Year Experience With High-Deductible Health Plans and Health Savings Accounts." Washington, D. C.: General Accountability Office, January 2006.

Geyman, John P., MD. "Family Practice in a Failing Health Care System: New Opportunities to Advocate for System Reform." *Journal of American Board of Family Practice* 15 (5) (2002): 407-16.

Geyman, John P., MD. "Myths as Barriers to Health Care Reform in the U.S." *International Journal of Health Services* 33 (2) (2003): 315-29.

Geyman, John P., MD. Myths and Memes About Single-Payer Health Insurance in the United States: A Rebuttal to Conservative Claims." *International Journal of Health Services* 35 (1) (2005): 63-90.

Glied, Sherry A. "Challenges and Options for Increasing the Number of Americans With Health Insurance." The Commonwealth Fund, January 2001.

Himmelstein, David U., MD; Steffie Woolhandler, MD, MPH; et al. "A National Health Program for the United States. A Physicians' Proposal." *New England Journal of Medicine* 320 (January 12, 1989): 102-08.

Himmelstein, David U., MD, and Steffie Woolhandler, MD, MPH. "National Health Insurance: Liberal Benefits, Conservative Spending." *Archives of Internal Medicine* 162 (May 13, 2002): 973-75.

Institute of Medicine. Committee on the Consequences of Uninsurance. *Insuring America's Health: Principles and Recommendations*. Washington, D. C.: National Academy Press, 2004, pp. 150-151.

Institute of Medicine. Committee on Educating Public Health Officials for the 21st Century. *Who Will Keep the Public Healthy? Educating Health Professionals for the 21st Century*. Washington, D. C.: National Academy Press, 2003.

Kahn, Charles N. III, and Ronald F. Pollack. "Building a Consensus for Expanding Health Coverage." *Health Affairs* 20 (1) (January/February 2001): 40-48.

Light, Donald W. "Health Care for All: A Conservative Case." *Commonweal* (February 22, 2002).

Meyer, Jack A., and Elliot K. Wicks. "Covering America. Real Remedies for the Uninsured." Economic and Social Research Institute, June 2001.

Nichols, L. M., P. B. Ginsburg, R. A. Berenson, J. Christianson, and R. C. Hurley. "Are Market Forces Strong Enough to Deliver Efficient Health Care Systems? Confidence Is Waning." *Health Affairs* (Millwood) 23 (2) (2004): 8-21.

Nyman, J. A. "Is 'Moral Hazard' Inefficient? The Policy Implications of a New Theory." *Health Affairs* (Millwood) 23 (5) (2004): 194-99.

Nyman, J. A. *The Theory of Demand for Health Insurance.* Stanford, CA: Stanford University Press, 2003.

Physicians for a National Health Program (PNHP) Web site: <www.pnhp.org>

"Proposal of the Physicians' Working Group for Single-Payer National Health Insurance." *JAMA* 290 (6) (August 13, 2003): 798-805. <www.physiciansproposal.org/proposal/Physicians%20ProposalJAMA.pdf>

The Future of Health Insurance in America

Fuchs, Victor R., PhD. "What's Ahead for Health Insurance in the United States?" *New England Journal of Medicine* 346 (23) (June 6, 2002): 1822-24.

"The Unraveling of Health Insurance." *Consumer Reports*, July 2002, pp. 48-53.

Public Health

Garrett, Laurie. *Betrayal of Trust: The Collapse of Global Public Health.* New York: Hyperion, 2000.

Public Perceptions

Graham Center One-Pager. "Who Will Have Health Insurance in 2025?" *American Family Physician* 72 (10) (2005): 1989.

Kaiser Family Foundation. "The Public on Health Care Costs: Perceived Reasons for Rising Health Care Costs." <http://www.kff.org/spotlight/healthcosts/index.cfm> (accessed May 25, 2006).

Schlesinger, M., S. Mitchell, and B. H. Gray. "Public Expectations of Nonprofit and For-Profit Ownership in American Medicine: Clarification and Implications." *Health Affairs* (Millwood) 23 (6) (2004): 181-91.

Schoen, C., S. K. How, I. Weinbaum, J. E. Craig, and K. Davis. "Public Views on Shaping the Future of the U. S. Health System." The Commonwealth Fund Commission on a High-Performance Health System, August 2006.

Wolfe, S. M., ed. "The People Have Spoken: The Drug Industry Doesn't Serve Us Well." *Health Letter*, Washington, D. C.: Public Citizen's Health Research Group. 20 (8) (2004): 1, 3.

Prevention (Obesity and Physical Activity)

Centers for Disease Control and Prevention. "Increasing Physical Activity: A Report on Recommendations of the Task Force on Community Preventive Services." In *MMWR (Morbidity and Mortality Weekly Report)* 50 (RR18;1) October 26, 2001.

Mokdad, Ali H., PhD, et al. "The Continuing Epidemics of Obesity and Diabetes in the United States." *JAMA* 286 (10) (September 12, 2001): 1195-1200.

Mokdad, Ali H., PhD, et al. "The Spread of the Obesity Epidemic in the United States, 1991-1998." *JAMA* 282 (16) (October 27, 1999): 1519-22.

Nelson, David E., et al. "State Trends in Health Risk Factors and Receipt of Clinical Preventive Services Among U.S. Adults During the 1990s." *JAMA* 287 (20) (May 22/29, 2002): 2659-67.

Nestle, Marion, PhD, MPH. *Food Politics. How the Food Industry Influences Nutrition and Health.* University of California Press, 2002.

Nestle, Marion, PhD, MPH, and Michael F. Jacobson, PhD. "Halting the Obesity Epidemic: A Public Health Policy Approach." *Public Health Reports* 115 (1) (January/February 2000): 12-24.

Schlosser, Eric. *Fast Food Nation: The Dark Side of the All-American Meal.* Boston: Houghton Mifflin, 2001.

Strauss, Richard S., MD, and Harold A. Pollack, PhD. "Epidemic Increase in Childhood Overweight, 1986-1998." *JAMA* 286 (22) (December 12, 2001): 2845-48.

Ethics in Health Care

Bekelman, J. E., Y. Li, and C. P. Gross. "Scope and Impact of Financial Conflicts of Interest in Biomedical Research: A Systematic Review." *JAMA* 289 (2003): 454-65.

Callahan, Daniel. *False Hopes.* New York: Simon & Schuster, 1998.

Geyman, John P., MD. *The Corporate Transformation of Health Care: Can the Public Interest Still Be Served?"* New York: Springer Publishing Company, 2004.

Kahn, C. N. "Intolerable Risk, Irreparable Harm: The Legacy of Physician-Owned Specialty Hospitals." *Health Affairs* (Millwood) 25 (1) (2006): 130-3.

Kassirer, J. P. *On the Take: How Medicine's Complicity With Big Business Can Endanger Your Health.* New York: Oxford University Press, 2005, p. 207.

Light, D. W. "The Practice and Ethics of Risk-Related Health Insurance." *JAMA* 267 (1992): 2503.

Medicare Payment Advisory Commission. "Report to the Congress: Physician-Owned Specialty Hospitals." Washington: MedPAC, March 8, 2005.

Pellegrino, E. D. "The Commodification of Medical and Health Care: The Moral Consequences of a Paradigm Shift from a Professional to a Market Ethic." *Journal of Medical Philosophy* 24 (1999): 243-66.

Pham, H. H., J. J. Devers, J. H. May, and R. Berenson. "Financial Pressures Spur Physician Entrepreneurialism." *Health Affairs* (Millwood) 23 (2) (2004): 70-81.

Reinhardt, Uwe E., PhD. "Wanted: A Clearly Articulated Social Ethic for American Health Care." *JAMA* 278 (17) (November 5, 1997): 1446-47.

Sider, Ronald J. "Does Justice Include Health Care for the Poor?" Chapter 6 in *Just Generosity. A New Vision for Overcoming Poverty in America.* Grand Rapids, MI: Baker Books, 1999.

The Medical Profession

Geyman, John P., MD. "Drawing on the Legacy of General Practice to Build the Future of Family Medicine." *Family Medicine* 36 (9) (2004): 631-8.

Stevens, R. A. "Public Roles for the Medical Profession in the United States: Beyond Theories of Decline and Fall." *Milbank Quarterly* 79 (3) (2001): 327.

Stevens, R. A. "Themes in the History of Medical Professionalism." *Mount Sinai Journal of Medicine* 69 (6) (2002): 362.

Fraud

Sparrow, Malcolm K. *License to Steal: How Fraud Bleeds America's Health Care System.* Westview Press, 2000.

Health Care in Other Countries

Anderson, Gerard, and Peter Sotir Hussey. "Comparing Health System Performance in OECD Countries." *Health Affairs* (May/June 2001).

Armstrong, Pat, and Hugh Armstrong, with Claudia Fegan, MD. *Universal Health Care: What the United States Can Learn From the Canadian Experience.* New York: The New Press, 1998.

Commission on the Future of Health Care in Canada <www.hc-sc.gc.ca/english/care/romanow/index1.html>

Organisation for Economic Co-operation and Development (OECD), Health Data 2001. See: <www.oecd.org>

Rice, Thomas, et al. "Special Section: Reconsidering the Role of Competition in Health Care Markets." *Journal of Health Politics, Policy, and Law* 25 (5) (October 2000): 863-978.

Saltman, Richard B., and Josep Figueras. "Analyzing the Evidence on European Health Care Reforms." *Health Affairs* 17 (2) (March/April 1998): 85-108.

Starfield, Barbara, MD, MPH. "Is U.S. Health Really the Best in the World?" *JAMA* 284 (4) (July 26, 2000): 483-85.

World Health Organization. *The World Health Report 2000. Health Systems: Improving Performance.* Geneva, 2000.

Medicare and Medicaid

Boccuti, C., and M. Moon. "Comparing Medicare and Private Insurers: Growth Rates in Spending Over Three Decades." *Health Affairs* (Millwood) 22 (2) (2003): 230.

Bodenheimer, T. "The Dismal Failures of Medicare Privatization." San Francisco: Senior Action Network, June 2003.

Commonwealth Fund. "MedPAC Votes to Urge Billions in Cuts to Private Plans in Medicare." *Health Policy Week*, April 25, 2005.

Dao, James. "On the Streets of Baltimore, the Word on Medicare Is 'Expand,' Not 'Reform.'" *The New York Times*, September 8, 2000.

Economic Policy Institute. *Paycheck Economics*. "Medicare at the Crossroads: Vouchers Take Us in the Wrong Direction." March 2001.

Geyman, John P., MD. *Shredding the Social Contract: The Privatization of Medicare*. Monroe, ME: Common Courage Press, 2006.

Kaiser Family Foundation Web site: <www.kff.org>

King, M., and M. Schlesinger, eds. *Final Report of the Study Panel on Medicare and Markets—The Role of Private Health Plans in Medicare: Lessons From the Past, Looking to the Future.*" Washington, D.C.: National Academy of Social Insurance, September, 2003, p. 28.

Public Citizen Report. "Medicare Privatization: The Case Against Relying on the HMOs and Private Insurers to Offer Prescription Drug Coverage, 2002." Available on the Web at <www.citizen.org/congress/reform/rx_benefits/drug_benefit/articles.cfm?ID-8298> (accessed October 2, 2003).

Health Care Costs, Co-Payments

Blumenthal, David, MD, MPP. "Controlling Health Care Expenditures." *New England Journal of Medicine* 344 (10) (March 8, 2001): 766-69.

Grumbach, K., and T. Bodenheimer. "Reins or Fences: A Physician's View of Cost Containment." *Health Affairs* (Millwood) 9 (1990): 120-6.

Kolata, Gina. "Medical Fees Are Often More for Uninsured." *The New York Times,* April 2, 2001.

Rasell, M. Edith, MD. "Cost Sharing in Health Insurance—a Reexamination." *New England Journal of Medicine* 332 (17) (April 27, 1995).

Tamblyn, R., R. Laprise, J. A. Hanley et al. "Adverse Effects Associated with Prescription Drug Cost-Sharing Among Poor and Elderly Persons." *JAMA* 285 (2001): 421-29.

Wielawski, Irene. "Gouging the Medically Uninsured: A Tale of Two Bills." *Health Affairs* 19 (5) (September/October 2000): 180-5.

Woolhandler, S., MD, MPH, and D. U. Himmelstein, MD. "Paying for National Health Insurance—and Not Getting It." *Health Affairs (Millwood)* 21 (4) (2002a): 88.

Woolhandler, S., MD, MPH, T. Campbell, MHA, and D. U. Himmelstein, MD. "Costs of Health Care Administration in the United States and Canada." *New England Journal of Medicine* 349 (August 21, 2003): 768-75.

Business and Health Care

Anthony, Joseph. "The Answer for Small Business: Guaranteed Health Care." December 2001. <Microsoft.bcentral.com/articles/Anthony/166>

Geyman, John P., MD. "The Corporate Transformation of Medicine and Its Impact on Costs and Access to Care." *Journal of American Board of Family Practice* 16 (2003): 443-54.

Gleckman, Howard. "The Nasty Side Effects of Medical Savings Accounts." *Business Week,* October 25, 1999, p. 42.

Kuttner, Robert. "A Dirty Little Secret: Managed Care Is Bad for Business." *Business Week*, December 21, 1998.

Kuttner, Robert. "The American Health Care System—Employer-Sponsored Health Coverage." *New England Journal of Medicine* 340 (3) (January 21, 1999): 248-52.

Kuttner, Robert. *Everything for Sale: The Virtues and Limits of Markets*. Chicago: University of Chicago Press, 1999.

Kuttner, Robert. "Must Good HMOs Go Bad? First of Two Parts: The Commercialism of Prepaid Group Health Care." *New England Journal of Medicine* 338 (1998): 1558-63.

Woolhandler, S., MD, and D. U. Himmelstein, MD. "When Money Is the Mission—The High Costs of Investor-Owned Care." *New England Journal of Medicine* 341 (1999): 444-46.

The Pharmaceutical Industry

Angell, Marcia, MD. "The Pharmaceutical Industry—to Whom Is It Accountable?" *New England Journal of Medicine* 342 (25) (June 22, 2000): 1902-04.

Angell, Marcia, MD, and A. S. Relman. "Prescription for Profit." www.washingtonpost.com. June 21, 2001.

Baker, D. "Patent Medicine." *The American Prospect*, January 29, 2001, pp. 34-35.

Bodenheimer, Thomas S., MD. "Affordable Prescriptions for the Elderly." *JAMA* 286 (14) (October 10, 2001): 1762-63.

General Accountability Office. "GAO Report Backs Link Between Drug User Fees and Higher Rate of Drug Withdrawals." *Health Letter* 18 (2002): 11.

Lexchin J., L. A. Bero, B. Djulbegovic, and O. Clark. "Pharmaceutical Industry Sponsorship and Research Outcome and Quality: A Systematic Review." *BMJ* 326 (2003): 1167.

Little, Shannon. "Public Citizen Report Debunks R&D Myths: Rx Drug Industry Exaggerates Costs, Blocks Efforts to Lower Drug Prices." *Public Citizen News* (September/October 2001): 4.

Lurie, P., C. M. Almeida, N. Stine, A. R. Stine, and S. M. Wolfe. "Financial Conflict of Interest and Voting Patterns at Food and Drug Administration Drug Advisory Committee Meetings." *JAMA* 295 (16) (2006): 1921-8.

Mueller, Rudolph J., MD. Chapter 4 in *As Sick as It Gets*. Dunkirk, NY: Olin Frederick, Inc., 2001. Web site: <www.nofreelunch.org>

Studdert, D. M., M. M. Mallo, and T. A. Brennan. "Financial Conflicts of Interest in Physicians' Relationships With the Pharmaceutical Industry—Self-Regulation in the Shadow of Federal Prosecution." *New England Journal of Medicine* 351 (18) (2004): 1891-1900.

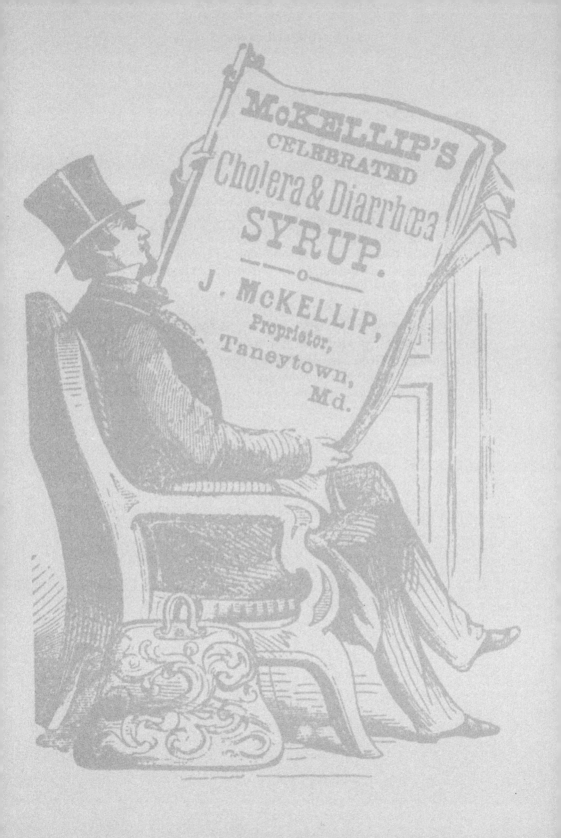

Appendix

Frequently Asked Questions (FAQs)
About "One Risk Pool"

Q. What defines "one risk pool"?

A risk pool is an insurance term used to describe a group of people who are all insured in the same group and, thus, share coverage and risk. The risk pool lumps them all together so no one person can be "wiped out" financially in case of a health catastrophe. Health care providers also are assured of payment. If there were "one risk pool" that included all 280 million people in America in the same group, the risk would be maximally shared. This would essentially constitute a form of national health insurance with universal coverage.

Q. Is "one risk pool" the same as "single payer"?

Not exactly, though it could be. "One risk pool" refers to the group of people—in this case, all Americans—enrolled in the plan. "Single payer" refers to a payment mechanism, where one entity, usually government, has the responsibility for paying the bills. It would be possible, though administratively more complex, to have multiple payers for a single risk pool.

Q. How is "one risk pool" similar to Medicare?

Medicare is a single risk pool for all Americans 65 years old and older (and a few other categories). For those 65 and over, the eligibility is universal and the enrollment automatic. In contrast, the proposed single risk pool includes everyone (all ages) in America. And the proposed single risk pool would have a more comprehensive range of benefits than the current Medicare.

Q. How would a "one risk pool" system be financed?

The overall financing would be similar to Medicare. But unlike traditional insurance (and to some extent Medicare) with its premiums, deductibles, and co-pays, the funding would come almost exclusively through progressive taxation, with everyone paying into a trust fund according to his/her ability to pay. It is not free.

Q. What is the role of government in the "one risk pool" approach?

Government would collect the taxes, assure the trust fund is solvent, oversee the system administratively, contract out for payments to providers, assure that guidelines are set for the benefit plan, and provide accountability to the American people for the functioning of the system. The delivery system would remain predominantly private, as is today.

Q. What would happen to the insurance companies under "one risk pool"?

The insurance companies would perform contracted administrative functions for the plan. They would be able to sell insurance for benefits not covered under the plan.

Q. What kind of benefit package would a system with "one risk pool" have?

It would be a comprehensive package, encompassing all "necessary" care, including inpatient and ambulatory care, emergency care, mental health, diagnostic testing, basic dental health, long-term care, eye care, and medical equipment. There would be no deductibles and no co-pays except for services deemed to be "marginal."

Q. Who would decide what the benefits would be with "one risk pool"?

The benefits package would be developed primarily through a consensus of the American people with the collaboration of "boards of health," both national and regional (or state). Priorities, guidelines, and global budgets will need to be set.

Q. How could such a generous benefit package be affordable with "one risk pool"?

"One risk pool" makes such a rich package affordable because of the vastly decreased administrative costs and the elimination of middlemen. These savings should amount to over $200 billion (2002 estimate)—more than enough to provide the resources needed to cover every person in America. Global budgeting helps to assure a cap on the spending.

Q. Wouldn't "choice" be decreased with "one risk pool"?

The opposite is true. There would in fact be more choice, as a person could go to any provider of his/her choice—including an HMO.

Q. Would someone be able to "opt out" of the pool and get "extra" care?

Hopefully, the "one risk pool" approach will be comprehensive enough and of high enough quality that there would be no need or desire to "opt out." However, anyone could buy supplemental insurance or pay out of pocket for services that are not covered. Beyond those limited circumstances, it will be up to the American people to decide whether to include "a safety valve" in the design of the plan—at the risk of creating a multitiered system.

Q. Would the "pool" include illegal immigrants?

A whole topic in itself. The short answer is "yes." These people do some of the most dangerous and difficult jobs in our society. They contribute more to our economy than they take out. And corporations that hire them often fail to provide them with health insurance, thus shifting the cost of their health care to taxpayers in general. The humanitarian answer is also "yes."

Q. Is it fair that someone who doesn't work and contribute to the trust fund gets a "free ride"?

The question reflects an "anti-welfare" sentiment expressed by many Americans. It brings into question the very existence of our current Medicaid program and ignores the fact that 80 percent of Americans who are uninsured are part of a working family. It also fails to recognize that everyone in America pays some taxes, be it sales tax, gasoline tax, or rent (which includes the landlord's real estate tax). And it overlooks the sad truth that many people are unable to work because of disabilities for which they're unable to get medical care. An example of "blaming the victim."

Q. What would we do with all the administrative people who would lose their jobs if we had a single risk pool? Wouldn't there be an economic disaster?

These people could be retrained to do useful work in the health care system, such as outreach, health education, and the provision of transportation. They would help meet the unmet needs. One example: nurses who now spend their time doing administrative work could once again do nursing.

Q. Isn't "one risk pool" the same as socialized medicine?

No. "One risk pool" is an insurance arrangement that allows huge administrative savings and enrollment equity—with everyone included and no one left out. The physicians and hospitals would be largely independent and not employed or owned by the government, as they are in the U.K., which has a system based primarily on socialized medicine.

Glossary

AAFP: American Academy of Family Physicians

ACP-ASIM: American College of Physicians/American Society of Internal Medicine. The specialists in internal medicine.

AHIP: America's Health Insurance Plans

AMA: American Medical Association

AMSA: American Medical Student Association

ANA: American Nurses Association

AHRQ: Agency for Healthcare Research and Quality

BBA: The Balanced Budget Amendment (1997)

CDC: Centers for Disease Control and Prevention

CHCs: Community Health Centers, a federally funded national program to expand access to care for poor and rural populations. They offer a sliding-fee scale for payment based on income, and are often referred to as "safety-net" clinics.

CHIP: See SCHIP.

CMS: Centers for Medicare & Medicaid Services; formerly HCFA (Health Care Financing Administration)

DRG: Diagnosis Related Groups, whereby a hospital is paid a set fee for a particular diagnosis

ER: Emergency Room

FPL: Federal Poverty Level

GAO: General Accountability Office

GDP: Gross Domestic Product

HCFA: Health Care Financing Administration; in 2001, renamed CMS (Centers for Medicare & Medicaid Services)

HHS: Health and Human Services

HIAA: Health Insurance Association of America

HMO: Health Maintenance Organization

HRSA: Health Resources Service Administration; a federal agency that is part of Health and Human Services

HSA: Health Savings Account (formerly Medical Savings Account)

JAMA: *Journal of the American Medical Association*

Medicaid: The federal/state health insurance program, initiated in 1965, that covers poor Americans, most nursing home costs, and a few other groups. Costs are shared between the federal and state governments. Eligibility varies from state to state.

Medicare: The federal health insurance program, also initiated in 1965, that covers people 65 and older, some disabled people, and people receiving renal dialysis

MRI scan: Magnetic Resonance Imagery, a relative of X-rays. It can be used to diagnose soft-tissue problems as well as abnormalities of bones.

MSA: Medical Savings Account (now called Health Savings Account)

NACHC: National Association of Community Health Centers

NHI: National Health Insurance

OECD: Organisation for Economic Co-operation and Development

PET scan: Positron Emission Tomography, a new and more expensive version of the MRI

PHS: Public Health Service

PNHP: Physicians for a National Health Program, a national organization, started in 1987, of more than 14,000 members advocating for single-payer national health insurance

PPO: Physician Provider Organization

R&D: Research and Development

SCHIP or CHIP: The (State) Children's Health Insurance Program, initiated in 1997, that expands coverage to near low-income children whose families earn too much for them to qualify for Medicaid. Some states have expanded SCHIP to include the parents.

UHCAN: Universal Health Coverage for America Network

USPSTF: U.S. Preventive Services Task Force

WHO: World Health Organization

Index

About the Authors

Bob LeBow, MD, MPH, was the Medical Director of a community health center in Idaho for over 25 years. A graduate of Harvard College and the Johns Hopkins School of Medicine, Dr. LeBow was board certified in two specialties: family practice and preventive medicine. He had extensive experience working on the development of health systems and preventive programs in over 20 developing countries, including a 2-year stint as a Peace Corps physician in Bolivia.

Dr. LeBow, however, devoted most of his career to addressing the problems of health care in the United States. A self-described "health care activist," in 1998 and 1999 he was president of Physicians for a National Health Program (PNHP).

He was paralyzed in a cycling accident in 2002 and died of complications from his injuries in late 2003.

C. Rocky White, MD, an internal medicine specialist, resides and practices in Alamosa, Colorado, where he also serves as the Medical Director for Cardio-Pulmonary Services at the San Luis Valley Regional Medical Center. He is currently the president of the San Luis Valley Medical Society, serves on the Colorado Medical Society's Leadership Committee and as a delegate to its Health Care Reform Congress, and also serves on U.S. Congressman John Salazar's Health Care Advisory Board. In addition, he is a former Medical Director for the San Luis Valley HMO. Dr. White has practiced rural medicine for the last 13 years. Raised in Nebraska, he attended Rhema Bible College in Tulsa, Oklahoma, and received his bachelor's from the University of Nebraska-Lincoln in 1987. He completed his Medical Doctorate and residency training at the University of Nebraska Medical Center and practiced in Sidney, Nebraska, for 2 years before moving to Alamosa. Dr. White, along with his wife, Debbie, and two daughters, Ariel and Aleeya, also farms and ranches in the San Luis Valley. He is a nationally known speaker and a strong proponent for major health care reform and has been active at the local, state, and national levels to effect change.